MCAD:
A Transport Guide to Mechanical & Circulatory Assist Devices

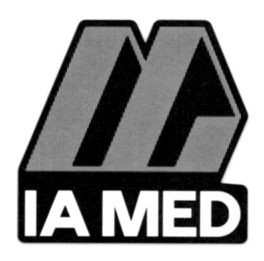

Dillon Wenberg, FP-C, CCP-C, CCEMT-P, NRP
Chris Smetana, AS, FP-C, CCP-C, NRP
Susie Smetana, MS, CCP

Editors

Tamas Alexy MD, PhD, FACC, FHFSA
Assistant Professor of Medicine, University of Minnesota
Advanced Heart Failure and Transplant Cardiology

Rishi Kumar MD
Assistant Professor, Department of Anesthesiology
Division of Cardiovascular Anesthesia
Division of Critical Care Medicine
UTHealth at McGovern Medical School

Aladdein Mattar MD
Assistant Professor of Surgery
Division of Cardiothoracic Transplantation and Circulatory Support
Baylor College of Medicine

Alexis Shafii MD
Associate Professor of Surgery
Baylor College of Medicine
Surgical Director Heart Transplantation

Education Committee
Chair - Jessica Peltz, BSN, RN, CFRN, EMT-P
Lead Registered Nurse - Jacob A. Miller, MS, APRN, FNP-BC, AGACNP-BC,
ACCNS-AG, CCRN, CFRN, NRP, FP-C
Lead Paramedic - Andy Fidino, NRP, FP-C
Lindsay V. Mauldin, RN, CFRN, CEN, NRP, FP-C, CCP-C
Tony Quesada

Medical Director
Mike Hudson, MD, EM, EMS
Air Medical Program Chief Medical Director
Level 1 ED Trauma Physician

Curriculum Designer
Jonathan Reed, BA, NRP, ATP, TP-C, FP-C, 18D

Cover / Graphic Designer
Mike Boone, BSN, RN, CFRN, CCRN

Reviewers
Brock Jenkins, FP-C, NRP
Allyson Moschera, NREMT-P
Jessica Peltz, BSN, RN, CFRN, EMT-P
Jeremy Singleton, RN, CEN
Dustin Stringham, MBA, NRP, FP-C

DISCLAIMER

The content, statements, views, and opinions herein are the sole expression of the respective authors and Immediate Action Medicine, INC.

The procedures and protocols in this book are based on the most current recommendations of responsible medical sources at the time of publication. Immediate Action Medicine, INC makes no guarantee as to and assumes no responsibility for, the correctness, sufficiency, or completeness of such information or recommendations. Other or additional safety measures may be required under particular circumstances.

This textbook is intended solely as a study guide to the appropriate procedures to be employed when rendering emergency care to the sick and injured. It is not intended as a standard of care required in an emergency, because circumstances and the patient's physical condition can widely vary from one emergency to another. It is not intended that this study guide shall, in any way, advise emergency personnel concerning legal authority to perform the activities or procedures discussed. Such local determination should be made only with the aid of legal counsel, your medical director, and your agency's protocols.

MCAD: A Transport Guide to Mechanical & Circulatory Assist Devices is an independent publication. It has not been authorized, sponsored, or otherwise approved by the owners of the trademarks or service marks referenced in this product.

Reference herein to any specific commercial product, process, or service by trade name, trademark, manufacturer, or otherwise does not constitute or imply its endorsement or recommendation by Immediate Action Medicine, INC, and such reference shall not be used for IA MED ©2020 *MCAD: A Transport Guide to Mechanical & Circulatory Assist Devices* study guide in advertising or product endorsement purposes. All trademarks displayed are the trademarks of the parties noted herein.

There may be images in this book that feature models; these models do not necessarily endorse, represent, or participate in the activities represented in the images. Any screenshots in this product are for educational and instructive purposes only. Any individuals and scenarios featured in the case studies or examples throughout this study guide may be real or fictitious but are used for instructional purposes only.

The QR Codes throughout the book are intended to be a quick link for readers to access videos and clips to aid the learning process as we know visualization is key to this new skill.

ISBN

9798574593141

Printed in the United States of America

DEDICATION

We want to dedicate the *MCAD: A Transport Guide to Mechanical & Circulatory Assist Devices* study guide and course to all of the students who are extending out of their comfort zone and striving to advance prehospital and critical care medicine.

This study guide was created to help cover the basic fundamentals of Mechanical & Circulatory Assist Devices in the pre-hospital (or prehospital) setting. It is our hope to elevate both the knowledge and the clinical confidence of the clinical provider through this text. We appreciate all the students who have provided us with continual feedback to improve our material and deliver both the knowledge and information they need to be successful as an advanced practicing medical clinician.

We would also like to thank all of IA MED's training partners throughout the United States and abroad for allowing us the opportunity to work with you in collaboration to help provide valuable education to your agencies and the communities you serve. We are truly honored and humbled to have been entrusted to do so.

ACKNOWLEDGEMENTS

I am humbled and thankful to have the support of my IA MED family who helped make this vision for the *MCAD: A Guide to Mechanical and Circulatory Assist Devices* course & study guide a reality. I hope that this guide can be used by anyone that operates in a critical care setting including air medical transport, ground critical care transport, and the CVICU. This guide is designed as a simple and easy to reference tool to both improve the confidence and the knowledge in the clinician using it. Our aim is also to improve the care rendered to patients that require these challenging devices.

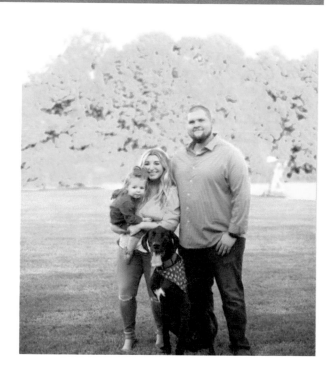

I would like to thank my mentors, and especially my close friends Chris Smetana and Mike Morrow. You guys always push me to succeed and operate out of my comfort zone and for that I am forever grateful.

Lastly I would like to thank my beautiful wife Taylor and daughter Charlie. Taylor you have always been my rock and encouraged me to dream big. Your support, love, and understanding throughout this long process of making this study guide possible has helped make this entire process enjoyable. You are the best wife and mother to our daughter that I could have ever asked for. I love you both more than words could ever say!

-Dillon

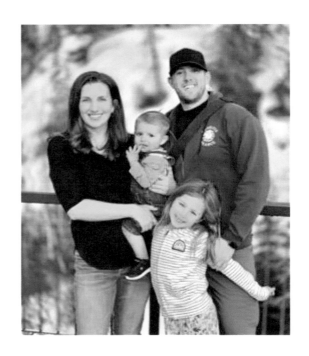

Susie and I personally would like to thank the IA MED Team for their continued hard work and selfless dedication to help IA MED become an industry leader in medical education.

We hope the MCAD study guide will help others continue to grow and understand the "why" behind these devices, making your next cardiac transport less intimidating and you a more confident and knowledgeable medical provider.

For the students who read this study guide, we hope the content inspires you. As you go out and practice, remember to always lead by example and help others learn along the way. Be that change in the industry and make an impact every day, no matter how small!

To our friends and business partner Jon & Kate, thank you for your support and the sacrifices you both have had to endure. "Ride or Die"

To our friends and family, thank you for all the help!

To our daughter, Shay, you are an amazing individual. We love all the smiles, laughter, and energy you bring to our lives. To our son, Ben, your kindness and empathy are a cornerstone of our family. As parents, we couldn't be more proud of your character and the individuals you are both growing into.

-Chris & Susie

PREFACE

Immediate Action Medicine, Inc. ("IA MED") is a disabled veteran-owned small business that provides cutting-edge specialty medical training, ranging from aeromedical critical care to austere tactical medicine. Our proprietary system has been continuously developed and refined since 2011, using a comprehensive data-driven approach.

MCAD: A Transport Guide to Mechanical & Circulatory Assist Devices is an addition to the IA MED education curriculum. It is designed to take the clinical provider to the next level of patient care and management.

Our unique approach to advanced medical education has made IA MED® the industry-standard and a fan-favorite among paramedics, nurses, and other industry providers.

MCAD: A Transport Guide to Mechanical & Circulatory Assist Devices will review the fundamentals of hemodynamics, art line management, ECMO, IMPELLA Support, LVAD, IABP and their transport considerations. The MCAD study guide will provide prehospital and critical care providers with a deeper understanding of the fundamental concepts of MCAD devices so they can apply them to clinical practice.

The intention of this book is not to make you a perfusionist but to provide a basic and introductory knowledge of MCAD.

Some sections below will provide you with QR codes to watch video clips for Impella, ECMO, and IABP support devices. Modern phones have a built in QR reader into the camera app or you can download a free QR reader.

This is EMS. Re-imagined.

TABLE OF CONTENTS

MCAD: A TRANSPORT GUIDE TO MECHANICAL & CIRCULATORY ASSIST DEVICES

Course Objectives:
- Discuss the principles of and indications for invasive hemodynamic monitoring
- Discuss indications, contraindications, and complications for arterial lines, central venous lines, balloon pumps, and other cardiac assist devices
- Describe general transport and flight considerations and troubleshooting common issues

WHY MCAD?

Applications:
- Decrease MVO2
- Improve coronary perfusion
- Improve oxygenation
- Decrease afterload
- Improve cardiac output
- Management of cardiogenic shock
- Improve MAP
- Improve end organ perfusion
- Improve right ventricular function
- Bridge to transplant
- Improve lung perfusion
- Heart recovery

Advantages:
- Portable
- Provides early stabilization
- Safe
- Allows recovery of vital organs
- Provides bridge to definitive care
- Guides clinical therapies

Disadvantages:
- Expensive
- Requires specialty training
- Can require additional personnel

ARTERIAL LINES

What is an Arterial Line?

An arterial line also known as an art-line, or a-line, consists of a thin plastic catheter inserted into an major artery. The art-line is most commonly used in perioperative and intensive care medicine to monitor blood pressure in real-time. Art-lines can also be utilized to obtain arterial blood gas samples for analysis.

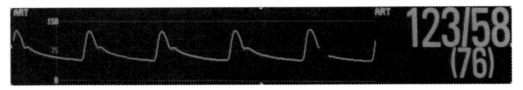

Why are Arterial Lines used in Critical Care transport?

Instant feedback

An art-line waveform is measured invasively (*inside the artery*) at the end of each heart beat and provides real time feedback of hemodynamic status, pharmacological interventions, and patient acuity. A non-invasive blood pressure (NIBP) measures at preset intervals and directly measure systolic and diastolic pressures. It also calculates mean arterial blood pressure (*MAP*), as well as heart rate.

The NIBP tracks the changes of systolic, diastolic, and mean blood pressure measured non-invasively on a preset set scheduled interval using a blood pressure cuff. To obtain the NIBP measurement the cuff inflates and deflates to measure both arterial occlusion and arterial pulsation.

The art-line performs in a similar manner by measuring systolic and diastolic blood pressures. It also calculates MAP, as well as heart rate, but in **real time** using a transducer via a cardiac monitor to provide a readable waveform.

This waveform is created by changes in vascular pressure that cause a pulsation of the saline column that is connected to the transducer. This moves the electromanometer's diaphragm. The diaphragm has a built in strain gauge. Deformation then causes a change in the resistance of the strain gauge. In simple terms, the transducer turns the pressure into a readable waveform.

https://litfl.com/arterial-line-and-pressure-transducer/

//► IA MED

Generally, arterial lines are not used to administer medication. This is due to the fact that many injectable drugs may lead to tissue damage that could possibly require amputation of the limb if administered into an artery.

Indications for Arterial Lines

- Hypotensive patients
- Serial ABG samples to track trends
- Can serve as alternate trigger source for IABP timing
- Patients on multiple vasoactive or antihypertensive medications

Setting up an Arterial Line

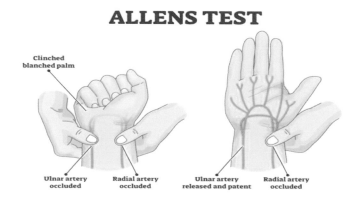

ALLENS TEST

Clinched blanched palm

Ulnar artery occluded

Radial artery occluded

Ulnar artery released and patent

Radial artery occluded

Prior to cannulation, an Allen's test should be completed. An Allen's test is performed by having the patient make multiple fists while the provider occludes both the radial and ulnar arteries. Once pressure is relieved to the ulnar artery the hand should return to a pink color. This reaction reveals that the ulnar artery creates enough perfusion to the patient's hand and an ART line can be placed.

However, if the patient's hand remains blanched for a prolonged period of time (> 5 seconds) when releasing pressure from the ulnar artery, this reveals the patient does not have enough collateral blood flow through the artery to sustain blood flow and perfusion. In this case, a peripheral ART line is not placed and other sites such as the femoral artery are considered. A pulse oximeter probe can be used to assess blood flow in patients that are sedated or unconscious. This will allow you to visualize the return of the pleth waveform at the time manual pressure is released.

Once cannulation of the artery is performed, connect the catheter to the rigid tubing and pressure-monitoring transducer.

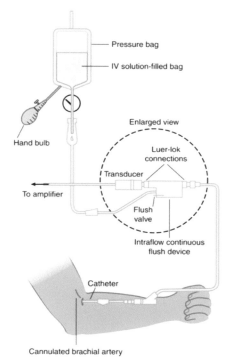

Pressure bag

IV solution-filled bag

Hand bulb

Enlarged view

Luer-lok connections

Transducer

To amplifier

Flush valve

Intraflow continuous flush device

Catheter

Cannulated brachial artery

Leveling the Transducer

Level the transducer at the Phelbostatic axis which is found at the 4 ICS, Midaxillary line.

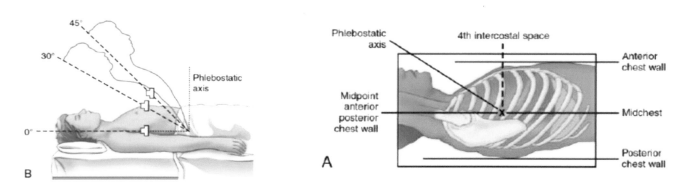

The most common cause of error in Arterial Line monitoring is **incorrect leveling of the transducer**

Zeroing the Transducer

1. Ensure the transducer tubing is correctly assembled and free of air bubbles
2. Place transducer at the phlebostatic axis
3. Turn the stopcock off to the patient and remove cap if needed
4. Press "zero" on monitor
5. Replace cap on transducer
6. Turn stopcock back on to the patient so it can monitor the pressure

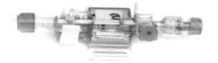

What does Zeroing the Arterial line do?

By Zeroing the arterial line at the correct position, the waveform has a true baseline of zero. This allows for the most accurate readings of real time blood pressure, including MAP.

The ART Line waveform

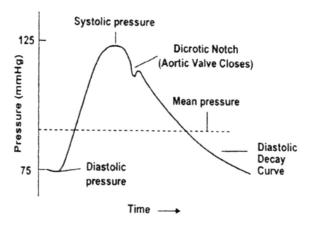

- Dicrotic notch represents Aortic Valve closure
- A Slurred dicrotic notch can represent a stenotic aortic valve
- The blood pressure in this example is 125/75.

Cardiac Transducer Troubleshooting

Fast Flush / Square wave test

Determines adequate dampening (assures proper pressure in the system)

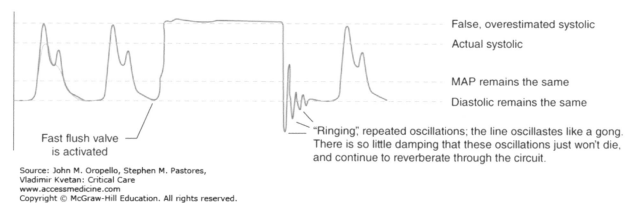

Source: John M. Oropello, Stephen M. Pastores, Vladimir Kvetan: Critical Care
www.accessmedicine.com
Copyright © McGraw-Hill Education. All rights reserved.

Arterial Line "Rule of 3's"

- 300 mmHg in pressure bag
- 3 ml/hr of fluid delivered into ART line
- Perform fast flush test for no more than 3 secs.
- Should see no more than 3 oscillations before returning to baseline

Cardiac Transducer Issues

Overdamping- system is not dynamic (too much pressure)

Pressure proximal to the transducer is too high causing pressure to over dominate the arterial pressure. Overestimates DBP and underestimates SBP.

Causes:
- "Overdamping = Obstruction"
  - Kinked line
  - Air in the line
  - Pressure bag overfilled
  - Boyles Law
  - Transducer placed too low

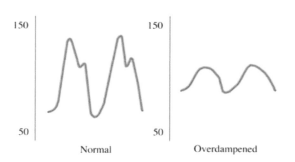

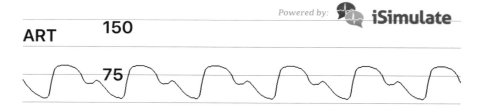

Underdamping - system is too dynamic (too little pressure)

Pressure proximal to the transducer is too low causing the arterial pressure to over dominate the pressure in the pressure bag. Overestimates SBP and underestimates DBP.

Causes:
- Pressure bag not full
- IV tubing is non-compliant
- Transducer placed too high

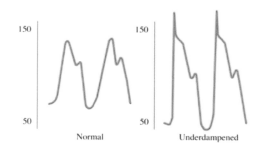

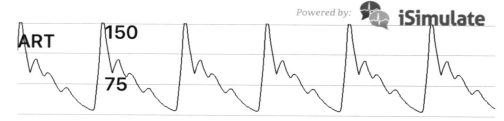

Central Venous Lines

A central venous line, or "central line" as they are most often called, are IV lines that are cannulated into central circulation.

A few examples of access sites include:

- Internal jugular veins
- Femoral veins
- Subclavian veins

Central venous lines can facilitate:

- Rapid fluid administration
- Medication administration
- Rapid access to central circulation
- Hemodynamic monitoring

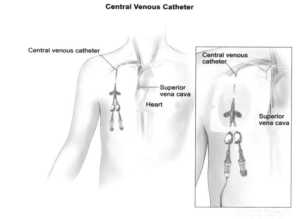

Central Venous Catheter

Central venous catheter

Superior vena cava

Heart

Central venous catheter

Superior vena cava

HEMODYNAMIC MONITORING

What is Hemodynamic Monitoring?

Hemodynamic monitoring records the blood pressure inside the veins, heart, and arteries. It also assesses blood flow and how well the body is oxygenating. It is a method to evaluate how well the heart is working.

Why is it important?

Hemodynamic monitoring provides a continuous assessment of the status of critically ill patients.

This can also show patient change in relation to ongoing therapies that are provided.

Hemodynamic monitoring can allow for a more accurate diagnosis and a quicker treatment plan specific to the diagnosis that is identified.

Pulmonary Artery Catheter/AKA Swan-Ganz Catheter

A pulmonary artery catheter is a multi-lumen catheter placed in pulmonary artery that allows for measurements of:

- Right heart preload (Central Venous Pressure)

- Right heart afterload (Pulmonary Vascular Resistance)
- Left heart preload (Pulmonary Artery Wedge Pressure)
- Cardiac Output
- Left heart afterload (Systemic Vascular Resistance)
- Core body temperature

The catheter is most commonly inserted into the subclavian vein or the internal jugular vein (https://youtu.be/ZBMhi5HrS2s)

The Catheter

The catheter ranges in size from 60 cm to 110 cm long.

Each small black line represents 10 cm with each bold black line representing 50 cm increments to help with insertion measurements of the catheter.

Each catheter consists of 4 lumens with thermodilution capabilities.

Proximal injectate port
- Used for monitoring **CVP/RA** pressure
- Provides cold thermodilution fluid
- Lumen is typically colored **Blue**

Thermodilution
- Uses an injection of cold fluid into the right atrium
- Cold fluid mixes with blood and drops the temperature cooling the blood
- The temperature is then measured again via the thermistor located at the end of the catheter in the pulmonary artery
- The rate of blood flow is inversely proportional to the change in temperature over time
- Uses the Hamilton-Stewart equation
- Used to measure the cardiac output

Proximal infusion port
- Used for rapid administration of fluid and medications

Pulmonary Artery distal lumen
- Used to obtain the measurements of **PA** pressure
- Also used for monitoring SVO2 measurements
- Lumen is typically **Yellow**

Balloon Lumen
- Inflates the balloon on the catheter
- Never to exceed 1.5 cc of air
- Allows for PAWP to be taken AKA "wedge pressure"
- Lumen is typically **Red**

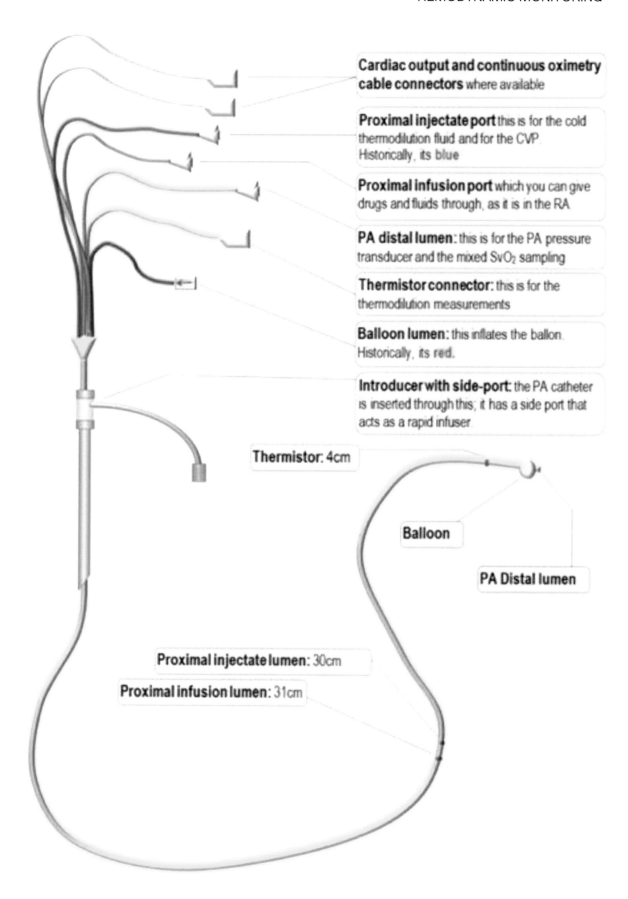

Cardiac output and continuous oximetry cable connectors where available

Proximal injectate port this is for the cold thermodilution fluid and for the CVP. Historically, its blue

Proximal infusion port which you can give drugs and fluids through, as it is in the RA.

PA distal lumen: this is for the PA pressure transducer and the mixed SvO$_2$ sampling

Thermistor connector: this is for the thermodilution measurements

Balloon lumen: this inflates the ballon. Historically, its red.

Introducer with side-port: the PA catheter is inserted through this; it has a side port that acts as a rapid infuser.

Thermistor: 4cm

Balloon

PA Distal lumen

Proximal injectate lumen: 30cm

Proximal infusion lumen: 31cm

Indications for Placement

- Hemodynamically unstable patients
- Patients suffering from severe shock
  - Cardiogenic
  - Neurogenic
  - Septic
  - Anaphylactic
  - Obstructive
  - Hypovolemic
- Patients receiving multiple vasoactive medications such as:
  - Inotropes
  - Vasopressors
  - Antihypertensive medications

Pulmonary Artery Catheter Placement and Progression Map

1. Passing through the Right Atrium (from the subclavian)
2. Passing into the Right Ventricle
3. Final destination, the Pulmonary Artery
4. Balloon inflated to get a "Wedge Pressure"

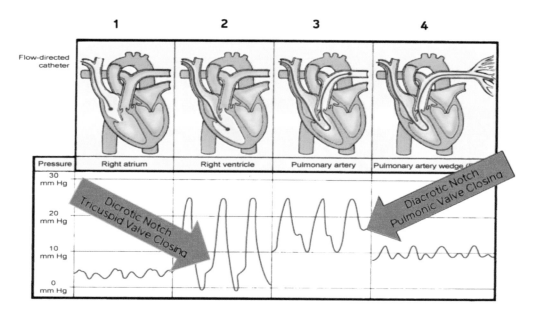

Dicrotic Notch on Left side of Waveform = RV Waveform (Tricuspid valve Closing)

Dicrotic Notch on Right side of Waveform = PA Waveform (Pulmonic valve Closing)

Pulmonary Artery Catheter Normal Values

Central Venous Pressure (CVP)
> **2 to 6 mmHg**
> Measures Right heart preload

Right Ventricular Pressure (RV)
> 15-25 mmHg systolic
> 0-5 mmHg diastolic

Pulmonary Artery Pressure (PA)
> **15-25 mmHg systolic**
> 8-15 mmHg diastolic

Pulmonary Artery Wedge Pressure (PAWP)
> **8-12 mmHg**
> Indirectly measures LVEDP (Left ventricular end diastolic pressure)
> Measures Left heart preload

Coronary Perfusion Pressure (CPP)
> **50-60 mmHg**
> DBP-PAWP

Cardiac Output (CO)
> 4-8 L/min

Cardiac Index (CI)
> 2.5-5.0 L/m

Systemic Vascular Resistance (SVR)
> 800-1200 dynes
> Left heart afterload
> > Resistance to flow in peripheral vasculature

Peripheral Vascular Resistance (PVR)
> 5—250 dynes
> Right heart afterload
> > Resistance to flow in pulmonary arteries

Mixed Venous Oxygen Saturation (SVO2)
Normal 60-80%

Mixed venous oxygen saturation (SvO2) is an indication of the percentage of oxygen bound to the hemoglobin once it has come back from arterial circulation returning to the right atrium. This is a reflection of the amount of oxygen that remains after the arterial side has utilized what it requires.

A decrease in SvO2 reveals an increase in oxygen demand for the body's tissues

    Hemodynamics Practice

https://abg.ninja/hemodynamics

Potential Complications Encountered During Transport

Migration of the catheter into the Right Ventricle

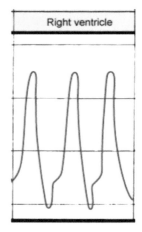

There are many reasons the catheter can migrate into the right ventricle. Most common being patient movement or transition from one cot to another etc.

The best way to identify if the catheter has migrated is to assess the PA waveform. If you note during assessment that the dicrotic notch is now located on the left side of the waveform (anacrotic notch) and the diastolic pressure has markedly decreased, chances are the catheter has migrated.

Migration of the catheter into the right ventricle can cause serious issues including ventricular arrhythmias. This is due to the tip of the catheter "whipping" around in the ventricle causing ventricular excitability.

It is **recommended** that in the event this happens in the transport environment, ensure the balloon is deflated and pull back on the PA catheter until a CVP waveform appears where your PA waveform would normally be. This ensures that the patient is safe and the catheter cannot cause further damage or ectopy.

IF you are utilizing this study guide as an aid for a higher level critical care exam. The procedure to replace the catheter back into the PA is as follows:

1. Inflate the cuff with **1.5** cc of <u>air</u>
2. Have the patient cough
3. Lay them on their right side

IA MED

Inadvertent Wedge Pressure (PAWP)

- Characterized by a wedge pressure waveform on the PA monitoring waveform
- The balloon is inadvertently inflated causing occlusion of blood flow in the pulmonary artery
- Can also be caused by catheter migration into the distal branch of the pulmonary artery
- This is the equivalent to giving the patient a pulmonary embolism!!

> ***This is life threatening and must be solved to ensure blood flow is restored to the pulmonary system.***

Procedure:

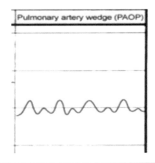

1. Ensure balloon is deflated
2. If possible have the patient cough
3. Patient positioning on left or right side
4. **Withdraw until you see a PA waveform**

> **A PAWP is typically not indicated during transport and can be estimated using the PADP (Pulmonary Artery Diastolic Pressure)**

Causes of Increased PA pressures

- Left ventricular failure
- Liver failure (portal hypertension)
- Cor Pulmonale (increased pulmonary vascular resistance)
- Mitral Regurgitation
- Mitral Stenosis

Pulmonary Artery Catheter PEARLS

- **Distal tip** is used to measure pressures
    - Do not exceed **1.5cc** air in distal cuff
    - Ensure the plunger on the syringe is completely depressed, ensuring no air is in the syringe. The stopcock is either open to the syringe in the event of residual air in the balloon or the stopcock is closed to the syringe, ensuring that there is no air in the balloon.
    - Do not take wedge pressure readings for **>15** seconds or **3** breaths
- Take readings at the **end of exhalation**
    - Equal pressure no active respiration occurring
- PA port only for **monitoring/lab sample** blood draw (not fluid resuscitation)
    - Use proximal port for infusions and fluid
- When transporting a patient with a PA catheter, deflate the balloon (prevents an inadvertent wedge pressure)
    - Balloon size increases at altitude due to **Boyle's Law**
    - The catheter may advance to an **inadvertent wedge**
- **Monitor for complications**
- **Catheter should be regularly exchanged every 14-30 days.**
    - Limiting the risk of infection

//⟋ IA MED

Hemodynamics in Shock

Type	Why?	Cause?	What happens?	Hemodynamic Changes?	Patient Presentation?
Hypovolemic	Loss of intravascular fluid volume	Hemorrhage Dehydration Burns	Decreased MAP due to volume loss	↓ CO/CI ↓ CVP ↓ PCWP ↑ SVR	↓ BP ↑ HR ↑ RR ↓ Urine output Cool, pale, moist skin Weak, thready pulse
Cardiogenic	Cardiac pump failure	MI Blunt chest trauma Dysrhythmia Structural defect Endocarditis Myocarditis Cardiomyopathy	Reduced contractility of the heart	↓ CO/CI ↑ CVP ↑ PCWP ↑ SVR	↓ BP ↑ HR ↑ RR + JVD ↓ Urine output ↓ LOC Cool, pale, moist skin

NORMAL HEMODYNAMIC VALUES							
CVP: 2-6	RV: SBP 15-25 DBP: 0-5	PA: SBP 15-25 DBP 8-15	PAWP: 8-12	CI: 2.5-5.0	CO: 4-8 L/m	SVR: 800-1200	PVR: 50-250

Type	Why?	Cause?	What happens?	Hemodynamic changes?	Patient presentation?
Obstructive	Circulatory collapse	Massive PE Tension Pneumothorax Cardiac Tamponade	Physical obstruction of circulatory intravascular blood volume leads to poor tissue perfusion	Dependent on etiology	↓ BP ↑ RR Chest pain/pressure Other symptoms dependent on etiology
Neurogenic	Loss of sympathetic nervous system tone	Injury to the spinal cord (common at C6 level and above)	Loss of spinal cord transmission causes loss of vascular tone	↓/normal CO/CI ↓/normal CVP ↓/normal PCWP ↓ SVR ↓ HR	↓ BP ↓ HR Cool, moist above Warm, dry below Diminished/absent motor/sensory function below injury

NORMAL HEMODYNAMIC VALUES							
CVP: 2-6	RV: SBP 15-25 DBP: 0-5	PA: SBP 15-25 DBP 8-15	PAWP: 8-12	CI: 2.5-5.0	CO: 4-8 L/m	SVR: 800-1200	PVR: 50-250

Type	Why?	Cause?	What happens?	Hemodynamic changes?	Patient presentation?
Septic	Decreased vascular tone and/or volume	Infection	Toxins and endotoxins enter system activating the SIRS response	Early ↑ CO/CI ↓/normal CVP ↓/normal PCWP ↓ SVR Late ↓ CO/CI ↓ CVP ↓ PCWP ↑ SVR	↓ BP ↑ HR ↑ RR ↑ Temperature ↓ Urine output ↓ LOC Bounding pulses Warm, flushed skin Petechiae Purpura
Anaphylactic	IgE mediated decrease in vascular tone and/or volume	Medications Insect bites/stings Envenomation Blood transfusion Imaging contrast Food	Chemical mediators released in response to allergy causing systemic vasodilation and capillary leaking	↑ CO/CI ↓ CVP ↓ PCWP ↓ SVR	↓ BP ↑ HR Shortness of breath Wheezing/stridor Pruritis/Urticaria Anxiety Flushed, red skin

NORMAL HEMODYNAMIC VALUES							
CVP: 2-6	RV: SBP 15-25 DBP: 0-5	PA: SBP 15-25 DBP 8-15	PAWP: 8-12	CI: 2.5-5.0	CO: 4-8 L/m	SVR: 800-1200	PVR: 50-250

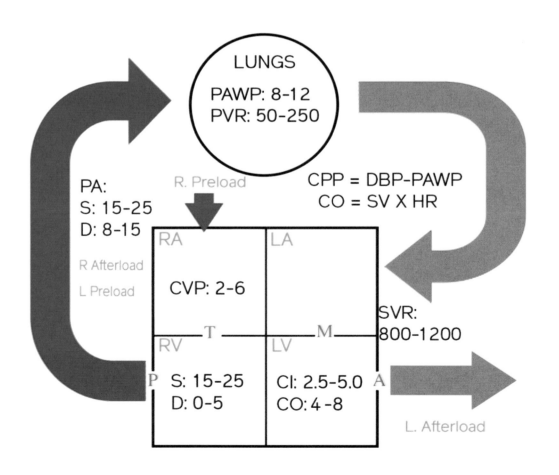

LUNGS
PAWP: 8-12
PVR: 50-250

PA:
S: 15-25
D: 8-15

R. Preload

CPP = DBP-PAWP
CO = SV X HR

RA   LA

R Afterload

L Preload

CVP: 2-6

SVR:
800-1200

RV   LV

T ——— M

P   S: 15-25   CI: 2.5-5.0   A
     D: 0-5   CO: 4-8

L. Afterload

INTRA-AORTIC BALLOON PUMP

What is an Intra-Aortic Balloon Pump

An IABP is a device that utilizes a balloon that is inserted through a catheter into a patient's aorta. The device is used to improve coronary perfusion pressure (CPP) and decrease workload on the heart by decreasing afterload. CPP is the amount of pressure to adequately perfuse the coronary arteries with oxygenated blood.

This is accomplished by inflation and deflation of the balloon at precisely timed intervals. The end result is an increase in aortic diastolic pressure and a decrease in afterload after systole (aortic end diastolic pressure).

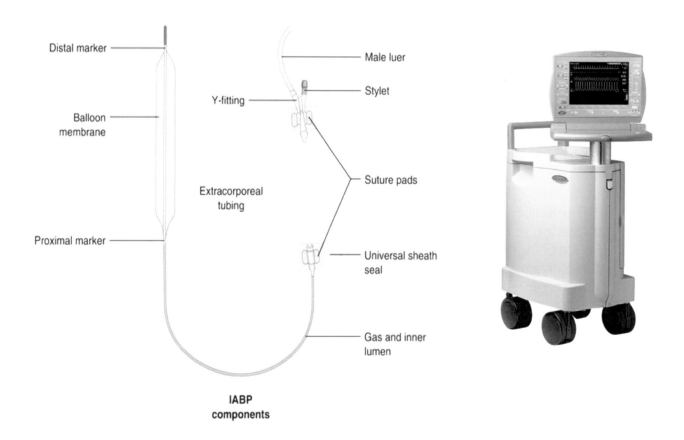

IABP
components

Inflation of the balloon upon the diastolic phase displaces blood flow under pressure back into the aortic root and coronary arteries. This improves the (CPP).

Deflation of the balloon just prior to systole drastically reduces the afterload that the left ventricle must overcome to eject blood and create forward flow. By reducing afterload there is a decrease of Myocardial Oxygen Consumption (MVO_2) and workload on the ventricle is dramatically reduced.

Indications for IABP Therapy

Acute Myocardial Infarction/Multi vessel occlusion
- Allows treatment to begin immediately by decreasing workload
    and improving coronary perfusion prior to receiving PCI

Cardiogenic shock
- Objective signs of shock
    - PAWP 18-20
    - Decreased UOP < 0.5 ml/kg/hr
    - SBP < 80 mmHg

Post CABG
- Allows the heart time to recover after open heart surgery
- Can be progressively weaned off of IABP therapy (ex) 1:1 -1:2 1:3 ratio

Contraindications

- Aortic Insufficiency (AI)/Disease
    - IABP inflation during diastole would worsen AI and force blood back into a recovering left ventricle
- Peripheral vascular disease (PVD)
    - Limb ischemia or known severe PVD
- Risk of rupture of vessels

IABP can cause a decrease in platelets (thrombocytopenia) due to hemolysis secondary to the balloon destroying RBCs upon inflation.

Effects of the IABP

- Improve Coronary Perfusion Pressure
  - Inflation
- Decrease workload (MVO$_2$) on the heart
  - Deflation
- Timing for the device is based upon ECG or pressure changes
  - Systole - IABP deflates
  - Diastole - IABP inflates

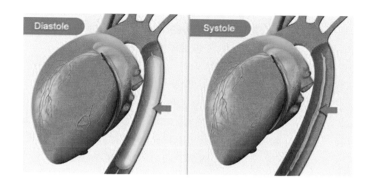

Placement of the IABP

The IABP is most commonly inserted through the femoral artery. However, some centers are beginning to insert the IABP via the subclavian artery. This site allows the patient to ambulate with the device still inserted and reduces possible deconditioning of the patient.

The final resting position of the IABP
- In the descending aorta
- 2-4 ICS mid clavicular
- Distal to the left subclavian artery
- Proximal to the renal arteries

Verifying placement of the IABP

The most definitive method for verifying the placement of the IABP is by utilizing a Chest X-Ray (CXR). When assessing the CXR. the radiopaque marker should be seen at the level of the 2-4 ICS midclavicular line (at the level of the carina).

However, if there is not a CXR available other reliable methods of placement verification can be used.

Check a left radial pulse
- Place the SpO2 on the patient's left hand
- If there is not an adequate pleth waveform or the pulses are not the same as the contralateral side, consider the balloon has migrated up and is occluding the left subclavian artery

Monitor UOP
- If urinary output is decreased consider that the balloon has migrated distally and is occluding the renal arteries.
- This will cause a decrease in UOP due to the decrease in renal perfusion.
  - Normal UOP for adults
    - 0.5/kg/hr OR 30-50 ml/hr

Components of the IABP Console

Trigger

The IABP trigger is just that. This is what source is selected to "trigger" or make the IABP balloon inflate and deflate.

The most common trigger is **ECG**. ECG uses the R wave to identify the beginning of systole.

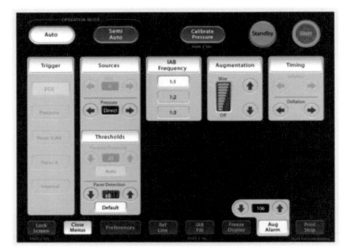

Touchscreen

Some balloon pump catheters have the ability to utilize a fiberoptic trigger. There is a pressure sensor located on the tip of the balloon itself and provides real-time aortic pressure waveforms and can be used as the trigger. Using fiberoptic trigger is "plug and play." Simply plug the orange cable into the fiberoptic port located on the balloon pump console and press "calibrate pressure" button on IABP keyboard.

In the event of arrhythmias and cardiac arrest, the trigger of choice is a **pressure waveform**. The pressure trigger works by using the ART line pressure waveform as an identifier of diastole. This is evidenced by the dicrotic notch symbolizing aortic valve closure.

Another trigger that is not utilized frequently is the **pacer trigger**. This utilizes pacing spikes to identify systole in the cardiac cycle. This mode is not as widely used due to the possibility of undersensing from the pacemaker causing R on T phenomenon. If the pacemaker is unable to capture, then the balloon pump will be unable to identify systole.

Shuttle tubing

The shuttle tubing is the plastic tubing that connects the IABP console to the IABP catheter. This shuttle tubing is what is responsible for carrying helium from the IABP console to the IABP upon inflation and deflation. It is important to monitor the shuttle tubing during transport or movement of the patient. Balloon migration is possible if the shuttle tubing is pulled on. If the shuttle tubing becomes disconnected, the IABP will be inoperable and alarm until the tubing is reconnected to the IABP device.

Ratio of augmentation

The ratio of augmentation simply means how many beats of the heart need to be augmented with the IABP device. For example, a patient that is critically ill and requires maximum support would be in a 1:1 ratio. This means that the IABP is augmenting with every beat of the heart. As the patient begins to improve you may then see that the ratio of augmentation is decreased to 1:2 or 1:3. This allows more of the native heart function to take over and only augments every other beat (1:2) or every third beat of the heart (1:3). You will commonly see this among patients that do not require as much support or their condition is beginning to improve.

"Auto vs Semi-Auto Operation Mode"

Think of auto operation mode as "autopilot". The console takes over and chooses what it believes is the most optimal inflation and deflation time. While in auto operation mode, you are unable to make any changes you see fit to the inflation and deflation timing. These settings will appear washed out on your IABP touch screen. In theory, auto sounds like a preferred operation mode, however, there is the potential for the patient to have a timing error and the console does not realize it. Semi-auto is a mode of operation that allows the provider to make changes to the inflation and deflation timing of the balloon. **You must be in semi-auto operation mode to make any changes to the IABP timing**.

How to Verify IABP Timing

Verifying correct timing of the inflation and deflation of the IABP is essential and must be monitored throughout the care of the patient. Timing errors can cause detrimental effects to the patient and if not caught can worsen the outcomes of IABP patients.

> **Remember you MUST be in at least a 1:2 ratio in order to properly verify timing of the IABP. This process cannot be done in a 1:1 ratio.**

Normal Timing

Decreases workload
Increases Coronary Perfusion

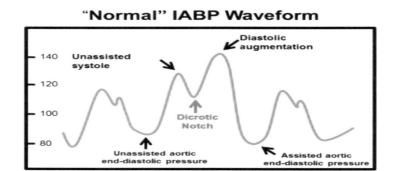

** Note the diastolic augmentation aortic pressure is greater than the unassisted systolic pressure. Also note that the assisted aortic end diastolic pressure is less than the unassisted aortic end diastolic pressure. These two key points tell us that the balloon waveform is normal. Inflation should occur almost even with the dicrotic notch and the dicrotic notch should not be seen in the inflation of the balloon. Deflation of the balloon should decrease the assisted aortic end diastolic pressure. If this is increased you have a timing error!

Inflation Timing Errors

Early Inflation

- The IABP inflates prior to aortic valve closing
- This process forces blood back into the left ventricle
    - Aortic Regurgitation
    - Decreased CO
    - Increased SVR
- Waveform appears to have a "U" shape
- Harmful to the patient

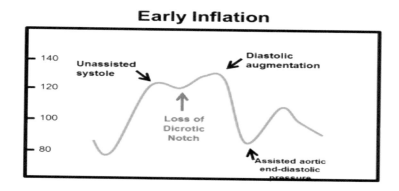

Late Inflation

- Inflation after aortic valve has already closed
- Not dangerous but sub therapeutic augmentation
- Decreased coronary perfusion
- "W" shape waveform

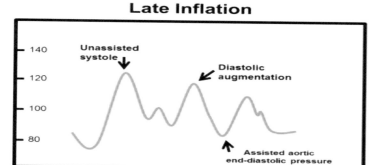

Deflation Timing Errors

Early Deflation

- Decreased negative pressure
- Increased afterload
- Deflation of balloon happens prior to systole
- "Cliff" shaped waveform

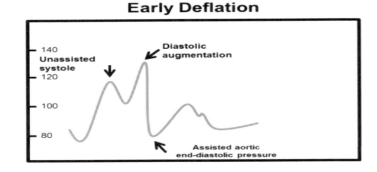

Late Deflation

- Increased workload on LV
- Increased afterload on LV
- Deflation of balloon happens during systole
- "Widened" appearance waveform
- HARMFUL

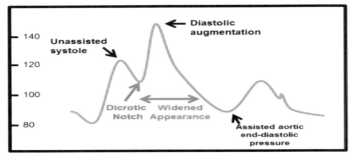

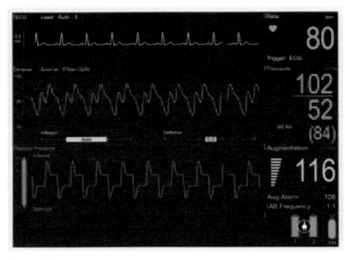

Monitor Display

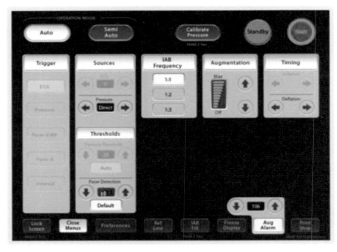

Touchscreen

IABP PEARLS For Transport

- Power failure
  - Manually pump every 3-5 minutes to prevent blood from clotting on the balloon
- There is no need to purge the IABP when going to altitude
  - The machine will purge itself
- Ensure you carry extra helium tanks prior to transport
  - It is bad form to run out while in flight
- If you see brown or rust colored flakes in IABP tubing
  - The tubing has ruptured the brown flakes are clotted RBCs inside the tubing system
- CPR
  - In the event the patient goes into cardiac arrest, switch the trigger on the IABP console to pressure by removing an EKG lead from the patient.
    - Most new machines will automatically switch to pressure trigger in the event of cardiac arrest.
  - Start chest compressions
- Battery
  - Keep the console plugged into A/C power whenever available to ensure the battery does not die
- Keep wires and connections loose
  - Pulling wires and shuttle tubing can cause disconnect from console or migration of the IABP
- Transport the console secured to an approved bracket
  - Ground or Air transport

IMPELLA

What is an Impella?

The Impella is a temporary Ventricular Assist Device on a catheter based platform. It can be inserted percutaneously or surgically into the left ventricle or pulmonary artery, depending on the support type desired. The catheter has a small axial motor that allows for suction of blood from the left ventricle to be displaced back into the Aorta. Unlike the IABP, the Impella pump is the world's smallest continuous heart pump. The catheter is designed to sit with the suction inlet in the left ventricle. The outlet port is designed to sit in the aorta. In the case of the Impella RP, the suction inlet lies in the left ventricle or vena cava and the outlet port lies in the pulmonary artery.

Impella Functions

- Temporary VAD
    - Typically not left in place more than two weeks
- World's smallest continuous flow heart pump (non-pulsatile)
- Offloads weak or failing left or right ventricle
- Boosts MAP and end organ perfusion
- Improves coronary and cerebral perfusion

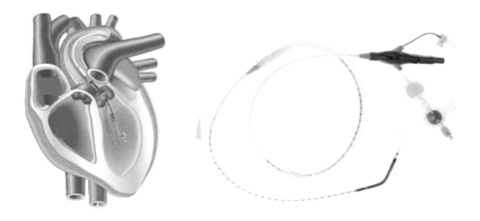

 Impella Introduction (with attention to soft keys)

https://www.youtube.com/watch?v=P3Plras_bjE

Impella Catheter sizes

Depending on the size of Impella chosen, the motor and catheter can augment up to 6.2 LPM (Impella 5.5) of cardiac output. The Impella RP is a right sided device that rests with the suction port in the inferior vena cava and the outlet in the PA. This allows for offloading of the right ventricle in the case of right sided heart failure or RVI.

Catheter Size	Flow Rate	Insertion Method
Impella 2.5	2.5 LPM	Percutaneous
Impella CP	3.5 LPM	Percutaneous
Impella 5.0	5.0 LPM	Surgically (cut down) Axillary
Impella 5.5	6.2 LPM	Surgically (cut down)
Impella LD	5.0 LPM	Surgically (cut down) Axillary
Impella RP	4.0 LPM	Percutaneous

Indications for Impella Therapy

- Heart Failure
- Cardiogenic shock
- High risk PCI
- Multi vessel occlusion
- Failure to wean from CBP
- Awaiting heart transplant
- Right ventricular failure

Contraindications for Impella Therapy

- Aortic Insufficiency
- Active hemorrhage
- Uncontrolled sepsis
- Left ventricular or atrial thrombi

Components of the Impella

Catheter / Motor

Impella CP® with SmartAssist® Pressure Sensing

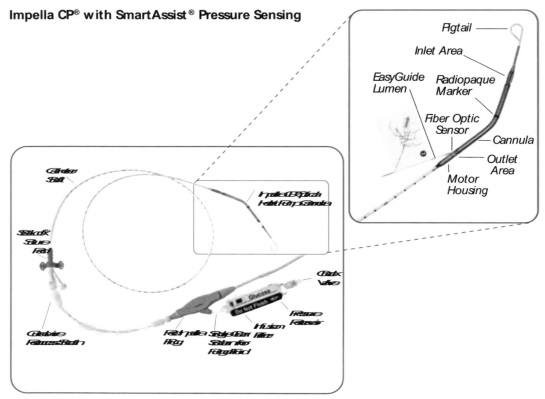

Impella CP with SmartAssist Clinical Reference Manual

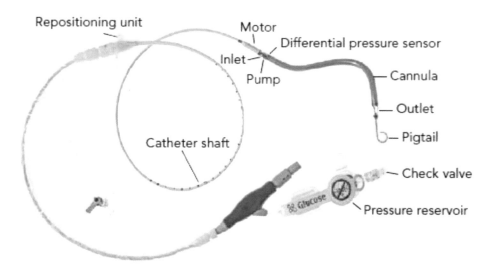

Impella RP with Automated Impella Controller Clinical Reference Manual

The plastic catheter is most commonly inserted into the femoral artery. Other sites of access can be axillary cut down, as well as surgically implanted. In the case of critical care transport, the preferred site will be the femoral artery via percutaneous insertion.

The most distal end of the catheter has a pigtail designed for stabilizing the device in the heart to prevent migration and ectopy. "Think of it like a boat rudder, keeping the ship straight in the current." The pigtail tip of the catheter could cause irritation of the ventricle in the event it touches the ventricular wall. <u>The Impella 5.5 does not have a pigtail.</u>

From the pigtail, the next landmark is the radiopaque marker utilized to assure the catheter is in the correct position. Next is the inlet area that is designed to allow suction of blood caused by the axial motor from the ventricle and force it under pressure through the outlet area located in the aorta. The outlet area of the catheter is located in the aorta or pulmonary artery, depending on catheter used (Impella RP). This is responsible for delivering the blood flow under pressure.

The housing for the motor is located just proximal to the outlet area and an open pressure port sits above the motor housing in the case of the Impella 2.5 and Impella CP. The Impella RP, LD, and 5.0 do not have the open pressure port on the catheter. This open pressure area is to gauge pressure changes from the LV to the Aorta or in the case of Impella RP the VC to the PA.

Another feature on the Impella catheter is the Touy Borst valve. It is located on the proximal end, where the catheter exits the patient. This colored plug connects the Arterial line pressure bag (2.5 and CP) as well as the purge fluid to the catheter. The purge fluid then is placed in the Impella console via the purge fluid cassette. The Touy Borst valve should be tightened down to secure the catheter in place. Take precaution to check the Touy Borst valve prior to transport to decrease risk of catheter migration.

Please note that placement of the catheter should take place under fluoroscopy and should not be repositioned unless done so by a physician.

Purge Fluid

Purge fluid is a mixture of Heparin 50 u/ml and Dextrose 5%-20% that is infused at a steady rate out of the Impella catheter. The main objective of purge fluid is to protect the motor. Dextrose is used because the fluid is viscous and can handle being pressurized. The dextrose fluid runs through the motor, and then comes out of the motor in the shape of a "V". This acts as a barrier for the motor housing and prevents blood from clotting in the motor. Blood clotting in the motor will cause device failure. The purge fluid is delivered and controlled by the Impella console via the purge cassette.

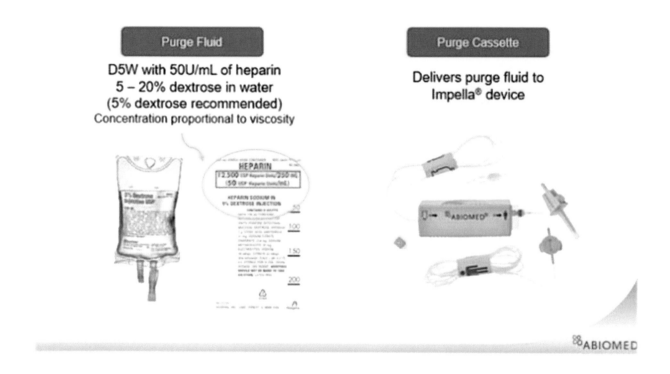

Console

This console is the actual monitor portion of the Impella device. The console weighs approximately 20 lbs. and must be secured to a mount if transported in an aircraft or ground MICU. The controller has various displays such as a summary, placement/waveform screen, and a purge fluid display. Often times, the screen is placed in the placement/waveform view. This allows the provider to see that the placement of the catheter is in an optimal position by utilizing the placement and motor current waveforms.

Soft Keys:

To the right hand side of the Impella screen you note soft keys. These soft keys provide various settings for the Impella controller.

Mute Alarm
Allows the controller to be muted when detecting alarms such as:
> Incorrect placement
> Purge fluid pressure low
> Purge fluid pressure high
> Suction

Flow Control or "P Level"
Allows the Power Level to be set on the Impella controller. The Power Level has settings from P-0 to P-8. The power level is set no lower than P-2 to prevent retrograde blood flow. Simply put, the higher the P level the more suction and greater augmentation of CO.

Display
Display controls which screen view is selected on the Impella controller.
Most often, the screen view that is most commonly used is the placement screen. The reason for this is that this display shows both waveforms for placement and motor current. Both of these waveforms are essential for verifying the Impella catheter is correctly positioned.

Other potential console views to note are the home screen and purge fluid screen. The home screen reveals a picture of the heart with the phrase Impella Position OK based upon the waveforms that the Impella console is seeing.

The purge fluid screen shows the total amount of fluid, dextrose, and Heparin that the patient has received each hour.

Purge Menu

Purge menu allows the provider to perform various tasks with purge fluid such as changing a bag of purge fluid, purging the system, changing the purge cassette, and de-airing the purge system.

Impella Flow

This is located in the bottom left hand corner of the Impella screen. It shows a small HUD of the mean Impella flow as well as the flows during systole and diastole.

Purge System

Purge system is located in the bottom middle section of the Impella screen. It shows the current purge pressure as well as the ml/hr flow of purge fluid.

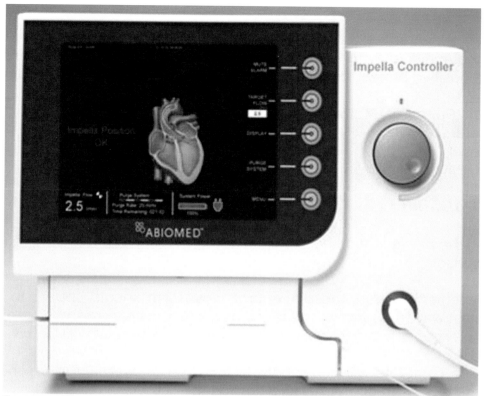

Summary View

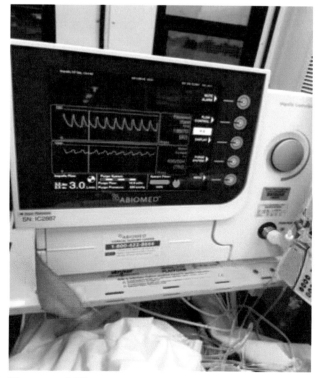

Placement View

Monitoring the Impella Device

It is important that multiple factors are monitored on the Impella device to ensure smooth operation and a positive benefit for the patient. To make this process easy, monitor the 4 P's of Impella:

Placement/Pulsatility (Motor Current)
Purge Fluid
Power Level
Pee... (UOP)

Placement / Pulsatility

When evaluating the placement of the Impella Catheter, it is important to be on the placement screen on the console.

Once at the placement screen, the **placement waveform** should appear to be aortic in nature. The easiest way to approach this is the placement waveform should look just like an **arterial line**. The exception to this rule is if the Impella catheter is an LD or 5.0.

In this case, these catheters will not appear to look like an arterial line on the placement screen due to the lack of an open pressure port on the catheter.

Just as important as the placement waveform is monitoring the **motor current waveform** for **pulsatility**. A pulsatile motor current reveals that the inlet and outlet ports are located in different areas of the heart (i.e.) LV and Aorta. In the case of a flat motor current, the inlet and outlet ports are in the same area of the heart and the catheter is misplaced or migrated.

Equally important, a flat motor current coupled with a flat placement waveform indicates that the patient is potentially pulseless and in cardiac arrest.

Note the difference in waveforms in the following imaging.

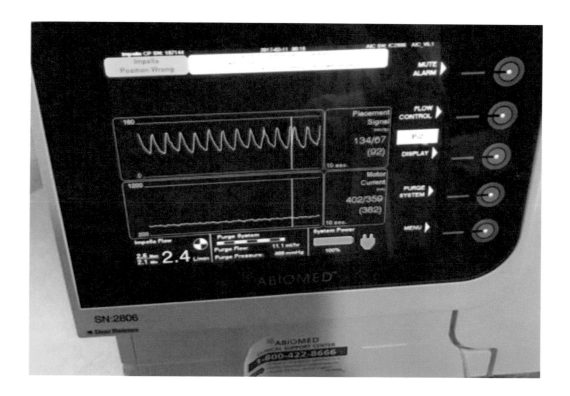

Note the "Impella Position Wrong" HUD. Also to note is the aortic appearing placement signal waveform and the flat motor current waveform (in green). This would indicate the catheter has migrated too far into the aorta and the inlet is no longer in the ventricle.

It is important to **treat the patient based upon their MAP not the reflected BP on the Impella console.** This is because the Impella catheter is not zeroed, which can lead to inaccuracy.

To verify MAP is accurate, obtain a manual BP cuff and use a doppler to verify the MAP matches the MAP on the Impella console.

Purge Fluid

Ensure that the provider is using the correct combination of Dextrose 5% - Dextrose 20% with 50 units/ml of Heparin added. Monitor the purge fluid HUD on the Impella screen to ensure that the **purge pressure** is between **300 and 1100 mmHg** and the ml/hr **purge fluid flow** is between **2-30 ml/hr** (per Abiomed guidelines). The Impella console should do this on its own.

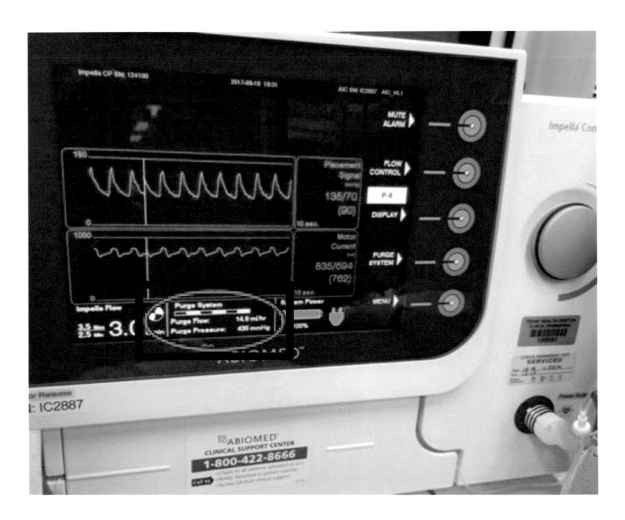

Power (P-Level)

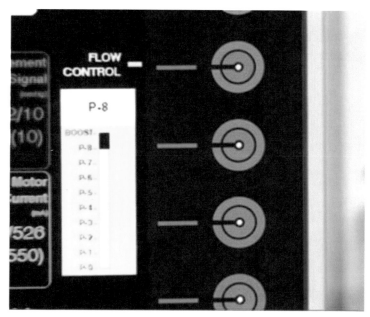

Power level is the setting that controls how much flow and CO you wish to augment.

P-2 is the lowest setting that should be utilized for a patient with a catheter still inserted. This setting is the minimum setting to prevent retrograde blood flow. P-8 is the highest setting that should be utilized. This is the power setting that will augment the most CO and cause the most flow.

The Flow Control menu on the Impella Controller

> **For patients on high flow levels, preload must be adequate. A target CVP of >10 mmHg is reasonable to ensure enough preload and prevent "suction" alarms from occurring on the Impella device.**

Urinary Output (Pee)

It is important to remember that the Impella device improves not only coronary perfusion, but overall MAP. With this in mind, renal perfusion is also improved and can lead to inadvertent diuresis.

Ensure an adequate urinary output of 30-50 ml/hr. This should be easy to accomplish due to the Impella improving renal perfusion and causing the kidneys to produce more urine.

Also, ensure that the patient continues to have adequate preload with a CVP of at least 10 mmHg. The Impella device is sensitive to volume and is preload dependent. Without adequate preload, the Impella will be unable to generate flows due lack of volume being available in the ventricle.

This will cause a suction alarm on the Impella console with a decrease in MAP and coronary perfusion pressure.

IMPELLA Flow Sheet

DATE: _____ Position (cm): _____ ABIOMED 1-800-422-8666

Time:	7	8	9	10	11	12	13	14	15	16	17	18	19	20	21	22	23	24	1	2	3	4	5	6
Mode: (Auto or P Level)																								
Flow: (L / min.)																								
Placement Signal: (Sys/Dia) mmHg																								
Motor Current: (Sys/Dia) Amp																								
Purge Pressure: (300-1100) mmHg																								
Purge Infusion Rate: (2-30 mL/hr)																								
Hep Infusion Rate: (Impella mL/hr)																								
Pump Position: (✓ or "OK")																								
Power: (AC / Battery)																								

Pump Serial Number: _____

Last Purge Cassette Change: _____

change every 72 hours

RN Name: _____   Signature: _____

AM LABS:

HCT: _____   HGB: _____

Platelets : _____   WBC: _____

PTT: ACT:

Time/Result: _____/_____   Time/Result: _____/_____

Time/Result: _____/_____   Time/Result: _____/_____

Time/Result: _____/_____   Time/Result: _____/_____

PATIENT LABEL

Example Impella Documentation Form

Common Impella Alarms

While managing a patient with an Impella, it is not uncommon to encounter alarms generated by the console. Below is a list of common alarms and complications that can occur while managing a patient on Impella support.

Impella Position Wrong / Incorrect Placement

Placement signal appears ventricular in nature
      Impella 2.5 and Impella CP
      Impella LD, 5.0, and RP have placement signal waveforms that do not appear aortic like
            the Impella CP and Impella 2.5

Motor Current waveform appears flat
      No pulsatile waveform

Potential causes of the alarm
      Catheter is too far in the Aorta
      Catheter is against the ventricular wall
      Cardiac arrest

Solution:
      Decrease power level to **P-2**
      Manage the patient pharmacologically
      Manage cardiac arrest etiology if applicable
      DO NOT try to replace or reposition catheter

Suction

Suction alarm is occurring due to lack of volume in the ventricle to create desired flow levels and CO. The ventricle collapses down upon itself due to lack of preload. This is also known as "suck down," or **"cavitating the pump."**

Potential causes:
> P-Level setting is set too high
> Preload is inadequate
>> Volume status (preload) is unable to keep up with desired flows
> *Obtain an ECHO to verify placement*

Solution:
> Administer volume to increase preload to ventricle
> Decrease the P-Level setting

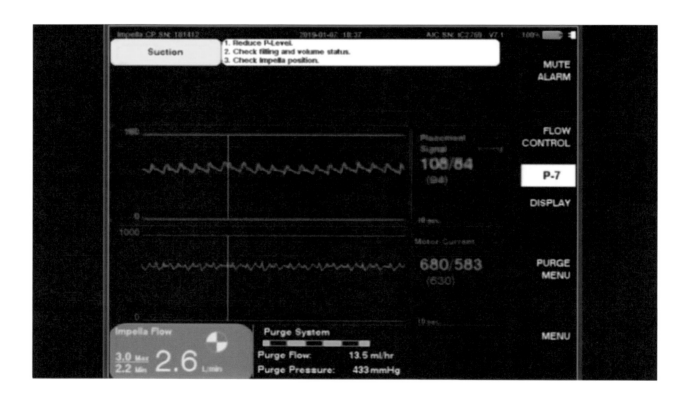

Low Purge Pressure

A low purge pressure alarm will sound when the Impella console senses that the purge pressure is below 300 mmHg

Potential causes:
> Concentration of Dextrose in purge fluid is too low
> Connections at the fittings of the catheter and purge cassette are loose

High Purge Pressure

A high purge pressure alarm will sound when the Impella console senses that the purge pressure is above 1100 mmHg.

Potential causes:
> Concentration of Dextrose in purge fluid is too high
> Tubing from purge fluid to Impella catheter has a kink in the tubing

Air in the Purge System

The Impella console has built in mechanisms to identify air in the purge tubing.

Potential Causes:
- Purge fluid bag was inverted during patient or equipment loading or moving
- Purge fluid is low in volume and requires a new bag

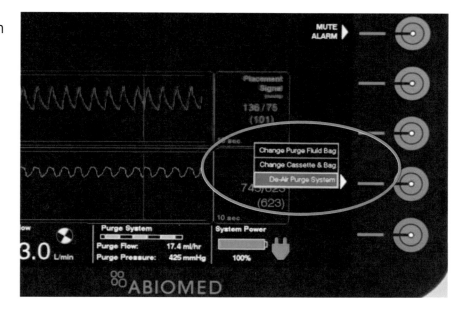

Solution:
- Use the "De Air tool" on the Impella console and follow prompts on screen to purge the system of air

Bleeding and Hemolysis

The Impella catheter has the potential to cause hemolysis if placement is incorrect or the catheter has migrated. This is more common the Impella 2.5 and Impella CP due to their smaller catheters having the ability to move and migrate more frequently.

During the assessment of an Impella patient:
    Assess the site for hematoma and bleeding
    If available, obtain a CBC to evaluate Hgb, Hct. Obtain ACT values.

If Hgb and Hct values are low
    Administer blood and/or platelets if warranted

If target ACT is low administer Heparin
    ACT target per Abiomed recommendation is 160-180

Safety and Transport PEARLS

The Impella console must be transported on an approved mount or securely in an aircraft or ambulance.

Console weighs 20 lbs.

Use the AC power cable when available to conserve battery power
    Battery power lasts for approximately 60 mins

Never increase the HOB greater than 30 degrees on a patient with an Impella catheter

Consider the use of a knee immobilizer to prevent the patient from bending / moving their lower extremity

Use care when moving or transferring a patient to prevent:
    Migration or dislodgement of the Impella catheter

Monitor pedal pulses with a doppler

Use of electrical therapy such as defibrillation, synchronized cardioversion and pacing is permitted

---

In the case of cardiac arrest, decrease the Power Level (P-Level) to P2 prior to initiating chest compressions

---

LEFT VENTRICULAR ASSIST DEVICE (LVAD) – LONG TERM

What is an LVAD?

An LVAD is a device that consists of an internally implanted pump. This device is designed to assume the gross majority of the left ventricular workload. This is accomplished by the implanted pump creating suction of blood from the left ventricle and displacing that blood into the Aorta under pressure. When this occurs. the MAP, coronary perfusion pressure and cerebral perfusion pressure are all increased.

LVAD Candidates

End-Stage Heart Failure

These devices are implanted for four main reasons:

Destination therapy:
> Designed to provide patients suffering from severe heart failure an improved quality of life.
>
> Heart transplantation is not considered due to the patient's wishes or the patient not meeting criteria to be considered for transplant.

Bridge to Transplant:
> The LVAD is placed in a patient suffering from severe heart failure to improve quality of life while awaiting a heart transplant donor.

Bridge to Decision:
> The patient receives an LVAD to improve quality of life while a decision is made regarding transplant candidacy.

Bridge to Recovery:
> This is most seen in short term VAD devices such as the Impella. The VAD is utilized to provide the heart with time to heal and improve from the pathology causing the severe heart failure if the cause is reversible.

Components of the LVAD

The long term LVAD device can be broken down into four major components: the implanted pump, the driveline, the controller, and the battery supply. All four major components must be in working order for the LVAD to function properly.

The pump

The LVAD pump is surgically implanted by a cardiothoracic (CT) surgeon.

The pump speed (RPM) is set during the implantation and is the only VAD parameter that can be directly adjusted on the console.

Pump inflow cannula:
    Creates suction of blood from the left ventricle
    Displaces blood into the pump

Pump outflow cannula:
    Returns blood from the LVAD pump to the Aorta under pressure
    Improves MAP, Coronary perfusion, and cerebral perfusion

Driveline

The driveline is a percutaneous cable that connects the external controller to the internally implanted pump. The driveline is responsible for sending a signal that allows the pump and controller to communicate and delivers electricity to the pump.

Be cautious not to fracture or cut the LVAD driveline. If the driveline develops a wire fracture or is cut for any reason, the LVAD will be inoperable and the patient will need to be managed aggressively.

LVAD Controller

The controller is a device that is worn externally on the patient. It is responsible for controlling the implanted pump. The controller can also monitor and reflect how well the LVAD is performing. The controller has a screen with a HUD that shows a variety of information such as: battery life, alarms, pump operation, and overall performance of the device.

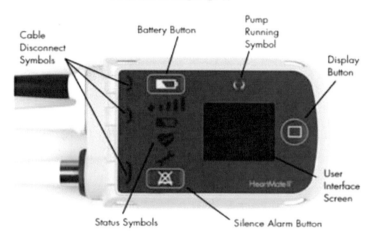

Controller from a HeartMate II LVAD

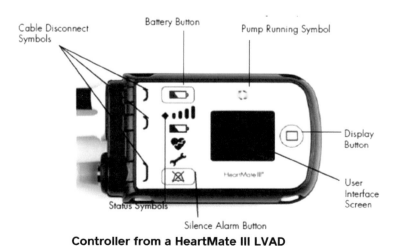

Controller from a HeartMate III LVAD

Battery / Power Supply

The battery supply is essential for the LVAD to operate. In a transport scenario, bring spare batteries and multiple power adapters in the event that transport is delayed.

 HeartMate 2 LVAD: Switching from used to charged batteries
https://www.youtube.com/watch?v=deJ3suKePAY

The LVAD has three power sources that the pump can utilize:

Battery Power:

> Batteries are rechargeable with a HUD to show battery life.

> **ALWAYS BRING EXTRA BATTERIES AND MULTIPLE POWER SOURCES FOR TRANSPORT!!**

A/C Power:

> Allows the patient to plug into a home outlet while sleeping. Also allows batteries to remain on the charger and recharge.

D/C Power:

> D/C power allows for adapters to allow the LVAD to charge via a vehicle charging portable charger.

Pulsatile vs Continuous Flow LVAD

Pulsatile Flow

The pulsatile flow LVAD is obsolete, is older technology and currently there are no living patients with the device. A pulsatile flow LVAD uses a pneumatic pump that has a collapsible chamber. The chamber fills with blood upon every beat of the heart. The pneumatic air then collapses the chamber filled with blood causing an augmented EF forcing blood into the ventricle. For example, this first generation LVAD is no longer used, it is an example of pulsatile flow.

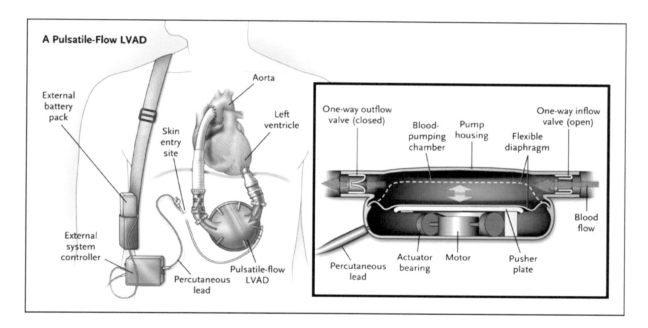

Limitations of the Device

Heart rate is set during implant of device and cannot be adjusted without another surgical procedure.

Cardiac Output depends upon:
- The set pump rate of the device
- Preload
- Afterload

Continuous Flow

All implanted LVADs today are continuous flow. With a continuous flow LVAD, an impeller continuously spins within the pump that creates suction from the LV and propels blood into the aorta under pressure. Example (HeartMate II, HeartMate III)

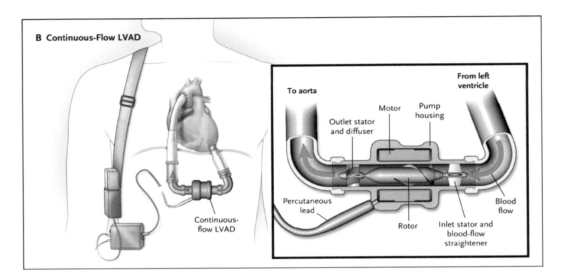

Limitations of the Device

Output of a continuous flow LVAD device is dependent upon:
- Set RPM (how fast the motor is set to spin)
- Preload (volume status)
- Afterload

> **If afterload is too high or preload is too low LVAD performance will decline.**

Assessment of the LVAD Patient

- Auscultation of the LV apex
  - Smooth "humming" sound should be noted
- It is common NOT to feel a palpable pulse (especially in continuous flow LVADs)
  - NIBP is highly unreliable and inaccurate this should NOT be utilized

> **Obtain hemodynamic status by assessing mental status and MAP.**
> **Utilize a manual cuff with doppler or an ART line if available.**

Potential Complications in LVAD Patients

Infection
- The leading cause of death in long term LVAD patients is sepsis
- Infection commonly occurs due to percutaneous driveline
- Treated with IV antibiotics (broad spectrum)
    - Septic shock management
- Often becomes a recurrent issue

Bleeding / Hemolysis
- Hemolysis is caused by destruction of RBCs as they travel through the VAD motor
    - Bleeding can be due to heavy anticoagulation therapies
    - Puts LVAD patients at risk for:
        - CVA
        - GI bleeding
        - Bleeding due to trauma/traumatic injuries
- Consideration to be made for patients that have a decreased MOI
- Treatment:
    - Volume replacement and blood as needed if hemorrhage is suspected.
    - Rapid transport to an LVAD capable trauma center is also indicated.

Thrombosis
- Caused by stagnant blood flow inside of the LVAD pump
- Blood coagulates and can create a thrombosis
- Treatment:
    - Thrombolytics
        - High risk for hemorrhage
    - Increased doses of patients anticoagulation medication

RV Dysfunction
- Due to the increase in flow from the LVAD, there is an increase in venous return that causes the right ventricle to see higher volume.
    - The right ventricle then dilates due to the higher volume which causes a decrease in contractile force
    - Septum shifts from right to left, due to lack of diastolic filling volume in the LV leading to further right ventricular dilation
    - Further right ventricular failure develops

Suck down Events
- Left Ventricle collapses due to lack of preload
- Can be attributed due to lack of preload to the left ventricle secondary to hypovolemia
  - Renal loss, GI loss, vomiting, dehydration
  - Also can be caused from RV dysfunction
- Can be characterized by a "knocking" sound heard upon auscultation of the LVAD

Treatment

Volume to increase preload to left ventricle. Inotropes to improve RV systolic function.

Device Failure
- If the device fails or the driveline is damaged this is an **EMERGENCY**
  - Requires rapid transport to the nearest LVAD capable facility
- LVAD may need to be replaced
- Mechanical failures are uncommon in the newest continuous flow LVADs (HeartMate III)
  - In the HeartMate III, all working components of the pump are held together by magnets
- Treatment:
  - Manage the patient pharmacologically and initiate rapid transport to LVAD facility
- If still unable to troubleshoot the device, call the LVAD coordinator. The number is often located on the back of the LVAD controller. They can assist with both equipment and clinical questions.
- **Electrical therapies are permissible if indicated**

CPR Considerations
- Chest compressions can cause cannulas to dislodge and internal bleeding to occur.
- Consider the following in the event a patient with an LVAD sustains cardiac arrest
  - Changing the controller, batteries, and power source
  - Administer a fluid bolus for volume replacement
  - Investigate and troubleshoot any alarms noted on the controller
- **If all is unsuccessful, CPR is the only chance at survival for the patient**

Troubleshooting LVAD Alarms

In the management and assessment of a patient with a long term implantable LVAD, it is not uncommon to note alarms for various reasons. The sound and color of the alarm are used to determine the severity of the issue encountered. The alarms are into two categories, yellow alarms and red alarms.

Yellow Alarms *(Advisory)*
- Illuminate a yellow light with an intermittent "beeping" sound
- Alarm is likely due to:
  - Low battery power
  - Cable is disconnected
  - Device malfunction

Red Alarms *(Critical / Hazard)*
- Illuminate a red light with one loud continuous tone
- These alarms indicate that the device needs immediate intervention
- Red alarms are often caused by the LVAD stopping operation or an issue with the Controller
- **Consider replacing the controller and immediately contacting the LVAD hotline on the back of the controller if the cause of the alarm has not been successfully determined**

Alarms Quick Reference:
https://qrgo.page.link/7exS2

HeartMate II LVAD Controller Alarms:
https://www.youtube.com/watch?v=7-Oypu1YCPw

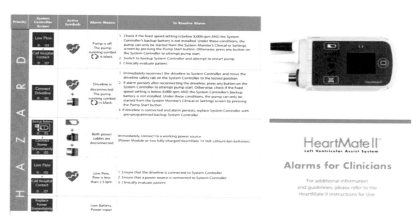

Example of a quick reference guide for the HeartMate II controller (Red Alarms), courtesy of HeartMate II

EXTRACORPOREAL MEMBRANE OXYGENATION (ECMO)

What is ECMO?

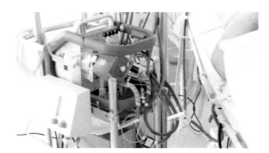

ECMO is an external device that is capable of oxygenating blood, diffusing CO_2, and augmenting cardiac output (depending on mode). You may have heard of this method of therapy described as a lung bypass or heart lung bypass (depending on the mode chosen). This therapy is reserved for critically ill patients that are unable to oxygenate using their own lungs and/or unable to adequately pump blood to the body due to heart dysfunction/failure.

The process is completed outside of the body prior to returning oxygenated blood back into the patient's circulatory system. To prevent hypothermia, the blood is also warmed via a heat exchanger before returning to the patients circulatory system. Depending on the mode used, the oxygenated blood can be returned to a venous site, an arterial site or both venous and arterial sites.

Since the first successful ECMO case was completed in 1971, the utility for ECMO in both prehospital and interfacility transport has largely been underutilized. Until recently, advances in both technology and size of equipment required to initiate therapy were limiting.

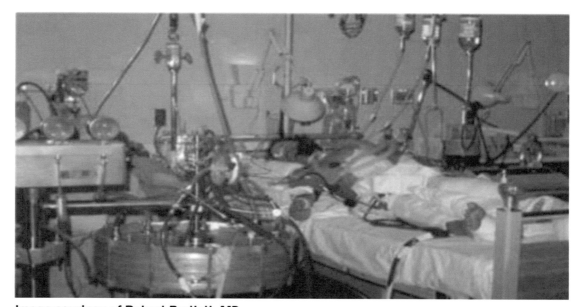

Image courtesy of Robert Bartlett, MD

Indications and Contraindications

 Extracorporeal Life Support Organization Criteria:

https://www.elso.org/Resources/Guidelines.aspx

Candidates for ECMO Therapy	
Cardiogenic Shock/MI	Hypothermia
Failure to wean from CBP	Post H/L transplant
Refractory Hypoxemia	Sepsis (rare)
ARDS	Certain Categories of Shock
Cardiac Arrest	Bridge to transplant
Drowning	

Contraindications for ECMO Therapy	
Unwitnessed Cardiac Arrest (prolonged downtime)	Severe COPD
Morbid Obesity	Advanced Age > 75
Active bleeding or infection	MODS
Terminal illness	

| Inclusion: | ECMO is indicated for **potentially reversible**, life-threatening forms of respiratory and / or cardiac failure which are unresponsive to conventional therapy | Or | Irreversible forms of cardiac or respiratory failure with option of VAD or Transplantation. (Age under 50) | TheAlfred |

| Exclusion (All forms ECMO): | Presence of additional severe chronic organ failure (liver, lung or renal)
Presence of severe acute brain injury
Malignancy
Age > 75 |

Exclusions for VA (Cardiac) ECMO Support:

Cardiac arrest: initial cardiac rhythm asystole or > 60 minutes to ROSC (or ECMO commencement)

Severe chronic pulmonary artery hypertension (even first presentation) with right ventricular failure and PAP$_{(sys)}$ > SBP

Un-repaired aortic dissection

Un-repaired moderate - severe aortic or mitral valve regurgitation with poor left ventricular function

Late Cardiogenic Shock - Process too advanced (≥ 3)

Lactate > 15

Advanced microcirculatory failure with severe mottling or established purpura

AST or ALT > 2000, or INR > 4.5

Anuria > 4 hours

Exclusions for VV (Respiratory) ECMO Support:

Irreversible process (ILD/pulmonary fibrosis, Bronchiolitis Obliterans, Cystic Fibrosis, Lung transplant > 30 days)

Immunosuppressed

(Other) Transplant recipients (heart, renal, bone marrow)

HIV-advanced

Advanced Septic shock - Process too advanced (≥ 3)

Lactate > 10

Noradren > 1.5µg/Kg/min

Severe myocardial depression

Advanced microcirculatory failure with severe mottling or established purpura

Image courtesy of Alfred ICU

IA MED

Modes of ECMO Therapy

The mode of ECMO chosen is the deciding factor if the machine is bypassing only the lungs for oxygenation and diffusion of CO_2 or *both* the heart and lungs with the added benefit of augmenting the cardiac output. If only the lungs are bypassed, this mode of therapy is dependent upon the patient's native heart function to pump the externally oxygenated blood from venous to systemic arterial circulation. In some cases, it may be necessary to return the externally oxygenated blood to both the arterial and venous circulation.

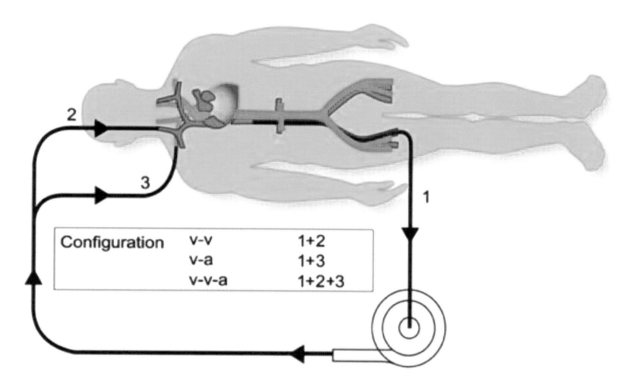

Configuration	v-v	1+2
	v-a	1+3
	v-v-a	1+2+3

Veno-Venous (VV) ECMO

In VV ECMO, blood is circulated from an inflow cannula that is placed at a venous site. Depending on the surgeon's preference, the site can be IJ, femoral vein, right atria, etc. Blood is then drained from the venous site via the cannula and travels through an oxygenator that oxygenates the blood and diffuses the CO2. The blood then travels through a pump and is warmed via a heat exchanger prior to returning to the body via an outflow cannula inserted in a different venous site.

Use of VV ECMO assumes the native heart function of the patient is adequate enough to assume all cardiac output. (Heart is responsible for pumping all of the externally oxygenated blood to arterial circulation).

VV ECMO can also act as a right ventricular assist device (RVAD) in the case that the right atrium and pulmonary artery are cannulated bypassing the right ventricle.

Avalon Catheter

An Avalon catheter is a type of catheter that is used in VV ECMO that allows for one cannulation site for both the inflow and outflow cannulas. The Avalon catheter is a dual lumen catheter that has the capability of suctioning blood from the IVC and SVC (inferior and superior vena cava) and delivering oxygenated blood directly into the heart via the right atrium. It is important that upon insertion into the IJ, the outlet port be directed towards the tricuspid valve. This is to prevent blood recirculation.

The benefit of the Avalon catheter is that the patient can ambulate preventing severe deconditioning. This also allows limited infection risk due to one cannulation site instead of two.

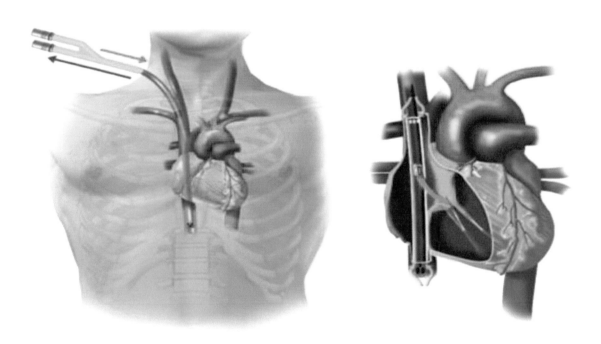

Blood is drained from the SVC & IVC and returned to the RA above the tricuspid valve

Veno-Arterial (VA) ECMO

In VA ECMO, blood is circulated from an inflow cannula that is placed at a venous site. Depending on the surgeon's preference, the site can be IJ, femoral vein, right atria, etc. Blood is then drained from the venous site via the cannula and travels through an oxygenator that oxygenates the blood and diffuses the CO_2. The blood then travels through a pump and is warmed via a heat exchanger prior to returning to the body via an outflow cannula inserted in an arterial site.

The ECMO pump can be used to augment cardiac output from 4-8 LPM of flow. This mode is reserved for patients with poor native heart function and the inability to oxygenate.

VA ECMO can not only oxygenate blood and diffuse CO_2, it can also reduce right heart preload and improve MAP due to the ECMO circuit providing a significant portion of the cardiac output.

EXTRACORPOREAL MEMBRANE OXYGENATION

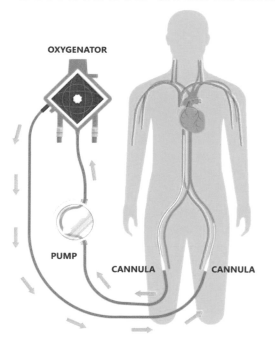

VENO-ARTERIAL (VA) ECMO

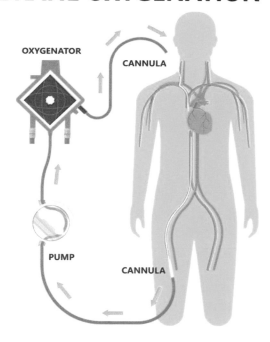

VENO-VENOUS (VV) ECMO

Veno-Arterial-Venous (VAV) ECMO

In VAV ECMO, blood is circulated from an inflow cannula that is placed at a venous site. Depending on the surgeon's preference, the site can be IJ, femoral vein, right atria, etc. Blood is then drained from the venous site via the cannula and travels through an oxygenator that oxygenates the blood and diffuses the CO_2. The blood then travels through a pump and is warmed via a heat exchanger prior to returning to the body via a bifurcated outflow cannula inserted in an arterial and venous site.

This configuration is often utilized in a case of peripheral VA ECMO with mixing cloud phenomenon (North vs South Syndrome) present.

North vs South Syndrome

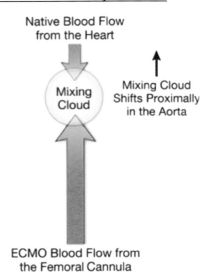

North vs South Syndrome (mixing cloud phenomenon) is characteristic of peripheral VA ECMO when upper extremity SpO2 is less than the lower extremity SpO2 with maxed ventilator settings. This is also referred to as **Harlequin Syndrome**.

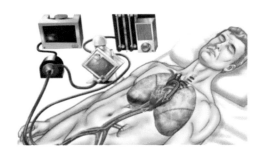

Poorly oxygenated blood from inadequately functioning lungs is returned into systemic circulation via native heart function This blood "mixes" with the rich oxygenated blood being returned to the arterial inflow cannula from the pump. The result is significant desaturation of blood in the upper extremities (where the two meet) greater than the lower extremities. This "cloud" of mixed oxygenated blood (native heart function vs ECMO rich oxygenated blood) can move depending upon the patient's heart function. For example, once the heart begins to recover, the EF will increase leading to more poorly oxygenated blood to move further down the descending aorta.

VAV ECMO used to boost oxygen content of blood coming into the RV prior to entering the lungs. This can also occur secondary to suction and inlet cannulas being too close together.

Always monitor patient ABG ad pulse oximeter from the right arm

This is most distal to arterial return and most reflective of coronary and cerebral oxygenation

ECMO+Impella (Ecpella)

In some cases it may be necessary to utilize Impella support in conjunction with VA ECMO.

Since the ECMO circuit cannot drain the venous system completely of the blood volume, fluid can still back up in the case of a patient with poor EF. The Impella is used to "vent the left ventricle" and displace the remaining backup of blood to the aorta, which is due to increased preload from the ECMO circuit. This also aids to prevent pulmonary vasculature congestion.

Components of ECMO

ECMO support utilizes four main components:
- Oxygenator
- Pump
- Heat Exchanger
- Inflow and Outflow cannulas

Oxygenator

An oxygenator is a dual chamber device that is separated by a semipermeable membrane.

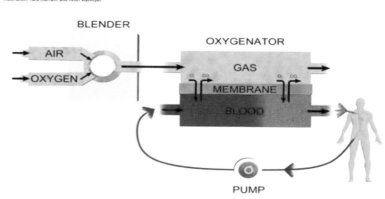

- Venous blood comes into one side of the oxygenator
- Sweep gas is delivered to the opposite side
- Gas exchange and dissipation of CO_2 takes place through the permeable membrane within the oxygenator.
- Causes uptake of oxygen and removal of CO2

Pump

The pump creates suction of venous blood into inlet cannula

After circulating through the oxygenator, the pump creates augmentation of CO and returns oxygenated blood back to venous or arterial circulation depending on ECMO mode. (VV or VA ECMO)

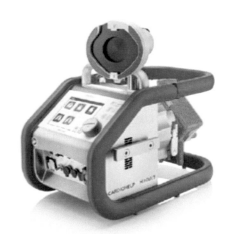

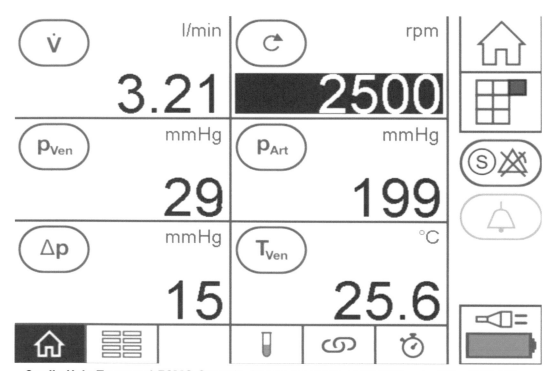

Cardio Help Transport ECMO Console, image courtesy of Rishi Kumar, MD of RK MD

For more information about the console, visit:

https://rk.md/2019/what-is-ecmo/

IA MED

Heat Exchanger & Cannulas

The heat exchanger is a device that ensures blood is warmed prior to returning into the body. This is to prevent hypothermia and its effects from occurring.

Cannula size is selected utilizing the formula **CI x BSA**. Muscle mass of patient is also taken into account to ensure metabolic oxygen demand is being met

> Inlet
>> Suction cannula (from venous)
>> Typically larger in diameter to facilitate better venous drainage
>> 22-28 French

> Outlet
>> Return cannula (to venous or arterial) depending on the mode selected
>> Typically smaller in diameter and shorter
>> 16-20 French

CRRT - Continuous Renal Replacement Therapy

> A form of hemodialysis that takes place over 24 hours
> Can be integrated with ECMO circuit to allow for dialysis while on ECMO

Patient must be Heparinized prior to cannula insertion with an ACT 220

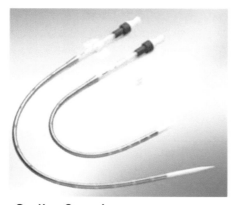

Suction Cannula

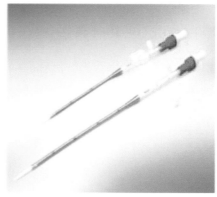

Return Cannula

Distal Perfusion Catheter

A distal perfusion cannula is a small catheter that bifurcates from the outlet cannula. The catheter is inserted towards the lower extremities to ensure lower extremities are perfused and lessens the risk of limb ischemia in peripheral ECMO configurations.

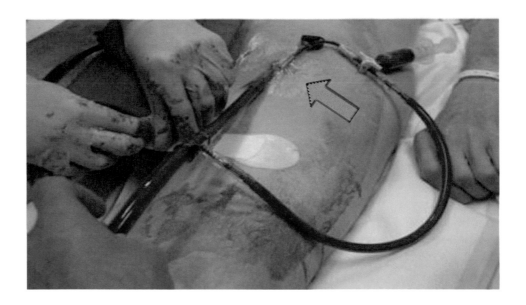

Oxygen

Oxygen is required for the oxygenator. A standard portable oxygen cylinder with a regulator is commonly all that is required for ECMO transport, as many programs do not have access to medical air.

ENSURE YOU DO NOT RUN OUT OF OXYGEN DURING TRANSPORT!!!

Potential Complications of ECMO Therapy

ECMO Complications	
Infection	Two direct routes directly into the body
Hemorrhage	Patients on anticoagulation therapy and Heparin (ACT 200-220)
Anemia	Caused from hemolysis due to motor
Thrombosis	Due to stagnant blood flow or air embolism from circuit
Death	Results from failure to wean from ECMO support (withdrawal)

Monitoring Considerations

Many factors must be monitored on a patient receiving ECMO therapy. The following are a list of common factors and settings that must be closely monitored. *This is not an all-inclusive list of everything to be monitored on an ECMO patient.*

Sweep

Sweep gas is delivered into the oxygenator using a combination of oxygen and medical air. If medical air is unavailable, only oxygen can be utilized.

> **The more sweep gas is utilized the more diffusion of CO_2 will take place.**

Increase the Sweep gas to lower CO_2 levels

Decrease the Sweep gas to allow CO_2 levels to rise

Fraction of Inspired Oxygen (FiO₂)

FiO₂ is required for the oxygenator and sweep gas to work effectively.

Room air oxygen is .21 and this can be titrated all the way to 1.0. It is recommended that 1.0 FiO2 be used for transport unless medical air is available for use.

Venous Pressure Drop

Venous pressure drop is the amount of decrease in venous pressure created from the suction cannula.

It is important not to exceed > 300 mmHg drop in venous pressure to prevent the ECMO pump from having a decrease in flow.

Assessment of the suction cannula circuit may reveal "line chatter," or vibration. This is due to the circuit collapsing down on itself secondary to lack of volume.

In the event this occurs, consider:

Hypovolemia

Flow is too high vs patient's volume status

There is a "kink" in the tubing or a clot has developed in the suction cannula causing a decrease in flow

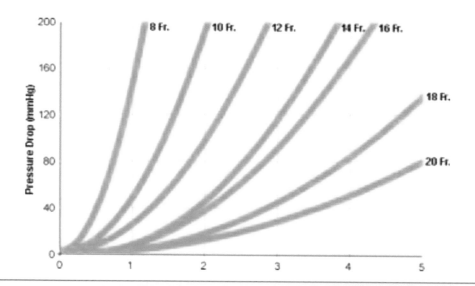

The smaller the cannula size the more venous pressure drop will occur.

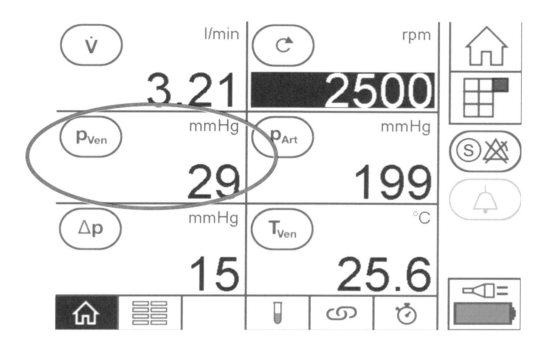

The venous pressure drop or Pven in this illustration is 29 mmHg

Treatment

> Administer volume
>
> Decrease flow on ECMO pump
>
> Consider blood products if hemoglobin is low. Consider the need to reposition the venous cannula upon arrival at the receiving facility.
>
> If third spacing is suspected administer 25% Albumin to maintain oncotic pressure

Condensation Buildup (Oxygenator)

In the event that condensation develops on the oxygenator, increase the oxygen via the regulator to 10-15 LPM flow.

This will blow off excess condensation that has built up over a prolonged period of time.

Utilize Safe Mechanical Ventilation

Prior to ECMO cannulation, many patients are on aggressive ventilator settings in an attempt to help the patient oxygenate. These aggressive maneuvers such as high levels of PEEP, inverse I:E ratio, APRV, Etc. can cause damage to the lungs resulting in barotrauma and possibly VILI.

Once the patient is cannulated onto ECMO, these aggressive settings are no longer needed due to the ECMO machines ability to oxygenate and diffuse CO_2 from outside of the body without use of the lungs.

It is important not to change the ventilator settings too drastically at one time. However an attempt at maintaining safe lung ventilation should be made in a stepwise fashion.

1. Lower the Vt or PC depending on the delivery chosen
2. Maintain a pPlat of < 27 if possible
3. If PaO2 remains low consider a blood transfusion if CBC (Hgb, Hct) is decreased.

Serial ABG Assessment

Serial ABG assessments are beneficial to identify if ECMO and ventilator therapy are adequate for the patient. The following is a brief synopsis for the possible acid/base disturbances identified with correlating treatments.

Oxygenation (PaO2)

In the case of a patient who appears to be hypoxic with an SpO2 < 95%, consider the following treatment methods.

- Increase RPM flows on the ECMO pump
  - Increases amount of oxygenated blood reaching the tissues and augments CO
- Utilize safe ventilation strategies
  - PEEP
  - Increase mean airway pressure
- Administer blood products
  - PRBC
  - FFP
  - Platelets if < 80k
- Ensure sedation is adequate

Respiratory Acidosis
      pH: <7.35
      PaCO2: > 45 mmHg

Consider increasing sweep gas into oxygenator to diffuse more CO_2

Utilize safe ventilation strategies (maintain safe lung ventilation)

Metabolic Acidosis
      pH: <7.35
      HCO3: <22 mmol/L

Increase RPM flow on ECMO

Increases more oxygenated blood to the tissues

Respiratory Alkalosis
      pH: >7.45
      PaCO2: < 35 mmHg

Decrease sweep gas on the oxygenator

      DO NOT turn sweep gas off completely

Metabolic Alkalosis
      pH: > 7.45
      HCO3: > 26 mmol/L

Commonly secondary to renal losses due to the increase in renal perfusion from the ECMO device.

      Consider administration of Lactated Ringers

Additional ABG Resources

 ABG Interpretation Practice with ABG Ninja

https://abg.ninja/abg

 IA MED ABG Module

https://training.iamed.us/courses/fmp-arterial-blood-gases

ECMO Transport PEARLS

Always carry a backup!!
    Cannulas, oxygenator, tubing, etc.
    In the event of power failure, utilize the hand crank.

Use a checklist to ensure you have everything you need
    Supplies, circuit, oxygenator, etc.

Maintain flows of at least 2LPM to prevent potential cause of blood clots

DO NOT exceed **37° C** on the heat exchanger

Monitor the oxygenator and tubing for potential clots hourly. If clots become worse and oxygenation continues to decrease, change the oxygenator

Never turn off sweep gas
    This will lead to respiratory acidosis

Do not decrease FiO_2 to a level that yields SpO2 < 95%

DO NOT RUSH

ECMO transport is NOT a fast process!!!

- Account for all slack in ECMO circuit
- Pay close attention to cannulation sites when turning or moving the patient to lessen chances of decannulation from occurring
- Secure the pump

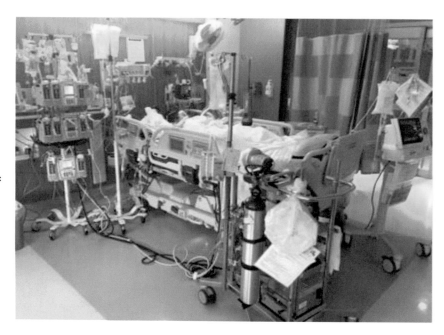

Potential Problems Encountered During Transport

Sudden Decannulation

A sudden decannulation from the ECMO circuit is a life threatening emergency that must be treated immediately.

The first action to be taken is to clamp and cut the distal ECMO cannula first.

> This prevents the ECMO circuit from continuing to expel blood from the cannula at the flow that is being utilized on the ECMO pump.

> Once the distal cannula is clamped, hold direct pressure on the site of decannulation

> Do not attempt to reinsert the cannula

> Immediate surgical intervention is indicated

Low SvO2 and SpO2

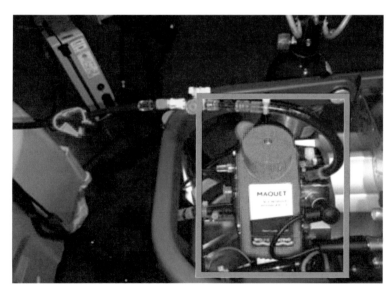

Mixed venous oxygen saturation (SvO2) is an indication of the percentage of oxygen bound to the hemoglobin once it has come back from arterial circulation returning to the right atrium. This is a reflection of the amount of oxygen that remains after the arterial side has utilized what it requires.

A decrease in SvO2 reveals an increase in oxygen demand for the body's tissues

Consider injecting into the PA catheter measurements as well.

In the event the SvO2 decreases < 60% consider:
　　Deep sedation
　　Maximizing RPM (flows) via ECMO to augment CO

A low SpO$_2$ can be caused due to the following:

- Poor placement of the SpO$_2$ probe
- Decrease in perfusion
  - Decreased flows via ECMO
    - Improve flows after ensuring adequate preload
  - Development of a clot in the circuit or oxygenator
  - Kink in the circuit tubing
    - Change the oxygenator / circuit tubing
  - Pulmonary edema
  - Fluid overload causing V/Q mismatch
    - Utilize PEEP on ventilator and diuretics if needed

Cardiac Arrest

VV ECMO

CPR IS necessary due to the arterial circulatory system not being augmented with oxygenated blood. VV ECMO depends on native heart function to distribute oxygenated blood to arterial circulation.

Electrical therapy is indicated.

VA ECMO

CPR IS NOT necessary as long as flow rates are adequate and sustain arterial oxygenation. Due to both the venous and arterial circulation being augmented and oxygenated by the oxygenator externally.

Electrical therapy is indicated.

Maximize flows on ECMO pump and consider POCUS to assess for cardiac activity

REVIEW QUESTIONS

1. When monitoring an ART line, the transducer should be zeroed at the:

   a. Foramen Magnum
   b. 4th ICS Mid Axillary
   c. 2-3 ICS Mid Clavicular
   d. 5th ICS Mid Axillary

2. Which of the following can cause overdampening of an arterial line waveform?

   a. Catheter Whip
   b. Hypothermia
   c. Pressure bag not full
   d. Pressure bag overfilled

3. A slurred dicrotic notch on an arterial line waveform is indicative of which of the following?

   a. Aortic valve stenosis
   b. Pulmonic valve regurgitation
   c. This is a normal finding
   d. Hypertension

4. As it relates to an arterial line, 300 mmHg in the pressure bag should deliver fluid into the artery at a rate of:

   a. 5 ml/hr
   b. 125 ml/hr
   c. 3 ml/hr
   d. 30 ml/hr

5. You are transporting a patient with the following arterial line waveform:

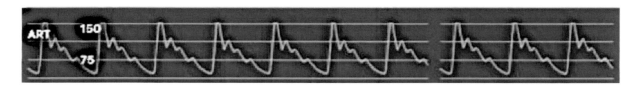

What abnormality if any is noted on the above tracing?
a. Overdamping
b. Oversensing
c. This tracing is a normal waveform
d. Underdamping

6. You have arrived on scene of an IFT to transport a patient with an arterial line. Upon your assessment, you are unsure if the arterial line MAP reading is accurate for the patient. What test if any can you complete to check the accuracy of the arterial line? [Select all that apply]

a. Flick test
b. Fast flush test
c. Square wave test
d. Transducer testing

7. An arterial line can serve as an alternative trigger source for which mechanical circulatory assist device?

a. IABP
b. ECMO
c. TAH
d. Impella

8. Which of the following can cause underdampening of an arterial line waveform?

a. Obstruction
b. Hypothermia
c. Kink in ART line tubing
d. An increase in altitude during transport

9. What does the dicrotic notch on the arterial line waveform symbolize?

    a. Opening of the aortic valve
    b. Pulmonic valve closure
    c. Closure of the aortic valve
    d. Mitral valve closure

10. You are transporting a patient with the following arterial line waveform:
What abnormality if any is noted on the above tracing?

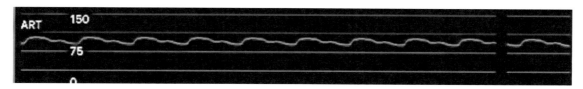

    a. Overdamping
    b. Underdamping
    c. Normal ART line waveform
    d. Pressure bag has less than 300 mmHg

11. You are assessing a male patient with a Swan Ganz catheter in place. You note the following hemodynamic values:

SVR: 1899 dynes   CVP 7 mmHg   PA: 34/22 mmHg
PAWP: 22 mmHg   CI: 1.9

Based on these values, what type of shock do you believe the patient is suffering from?

    a. Neurological Shock
    b. Anaphylactic Shock
    c. Cardiogenic Shock
    d. Right Ventricular MI

12. You are transporting a female patient from an outlying rural facility. A Swan Ganz catheter is in place with the following hemodynamic values:

SVR: 1799 dynes   CVP 0 mmHg   PA: 12/7 mmHg
PAWP: 2 mmHg   CI: 1.8

Based on these values, which of the following therapies would this patient most benefit from?

    a. Phenylephrine
    b. Dobutamine
    c. Whole Blood
    d. Nitroglycerine

13. You are transporting a female patient from an outlying PCI capable facility. You note the patient has a Swan Ganz catheter in place with the following hemodynamic values:

SVR: 1899 dynes   CVP 12 mmHg   PA: 34/22 mmHg
PAWP: 5 mmHg   CI: 1.9

Based on these values, which of the following types of shock do you believe the patient is suffering from?.

    a. Obstructive Shock
    b. Septic Shock
    c. Cardiogenic Shock
    d. Neurogenic Shock

14. You are called to an IFT for a female patient who has a Swan Ganz catheter in place. You note the following hemodynamic values:

SVR: 400 dynes   CVP 1 mmHg   PA: 14/8 mmHg
PAWP: 2 mmHg   CI: 1.3

Based on these values, which of the following shocks is the patient likely suffering from?

    a. Obstructive
    b. Hypovolemic
    c. Neurogenic
    d. Cardiogenic

15. You are transporting a male patient from an outlying rural facility. According to report, the patient has been intubated and on a ventilator for 7 days. Over the last 24 hours the patient has become more hypoxic with a PIP of 45 and pPlat of 36. A Swan Ganz catheter in place with the following hemodynamic values:

SVR: 650 dynes   CVP 1 mmHg   PA: 38/24 mmHg
PAWP: 16 mmHg   CI: 5.3

Based on these values, which therapy would the patient likely benefit from the most?

    a. Dobutamine
    b. Norepinephrine
    c. Milrinone
    d. Nitroprusside

16. You are transporting a female patient from an outlying PCI capable facility. While in the cath lab, a Swan Ganz catheter was placed with the following hemodynamic values:

SVR: 1950 dynes   CVP 11 mmHg   PA: 13/5 mmHg
PAWP: 6 mmHg   CI: 1.7

Based on these values, what is the patient most likely suffering from?

    a. Right Ventricular MI
    b. Left Ventricular MI
    c. Anaphylactic Shock
    d. Hemorrhage

17. You arrive at an IFT of a 69/F patient. You note upon your assessment that the patient has a Swan Ganz catheter. Given your knowledge about this catheter you know a PAWP should only be taken: [Select all that apply]

    a. At the end of exhalation
    b. No longer than 15 seconds
    c. No longer than 3 breaths
    d. No longer than 30 seconds

18. Upon arrival of an ICU transport, you note your patient has an intact Swan Ganz catheter. Upon moving the patient to your cot, you notice the patient has now what appears to be VT on the cardiac monitor. What should be your first course of action?

    a. Administer Epinephrine
    b. Start CPR
    c. Check for catheter migration
    d. Defibrillate the patient

19. While monitoring a Swan Ganz catheter what waveform MUST be continuously monitored if your equipment only allows for monitoring of ONE waveform tracing?

    a. CVP
    b. PA
    c. RV
    d. PAWP

20. As it relates to hemodynamic monitoring the PAWP is an indirect measurement of the:

    a. SV
    b. SVR
    c. PVR
    d. LVEDP

21. Which of the following would cause an increase in PA pressure?

    a. Tricuspid valve regurgitation
    b. Pulmonic valve stenosis
    c. Mitral valve stenosis
    d. Respiratory Alkalosis

22. What is the deadliest IABP timing error?

    a. Late Deflation
    b. Early Deflation
    c. Late Inflation
    d. Late Deflation

23. Inflation of the IABP balloon promotes:

    a. Afterload reduction
    b. Pulsatility
    c. Coronary artery perfusion
    d. Vasoconstriciton

24. Identify the IABP timing error:

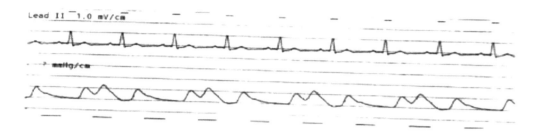

    a. Early Deflation
    b. Early Inflation
    c. Late Inflation
    d. Late Deflation

25. Identify the IABP timing error:

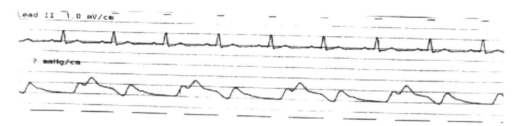

    a. Late Deflation
    b. Early Inflation
    c. Late Inflation
    d. Early Deflation

26. Identify the IABP timing error:

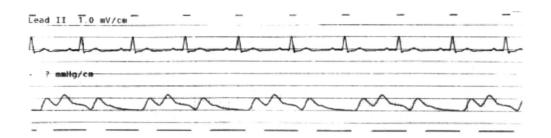

a. Early Inflation
b. Early Deflation
c. Late Inflation
d. Late Deflation

27. Deflation of the IABP balloon promotes:

a. Coronary artery perfusion
b. Sweep
c. Afterload reduction
d. Increase in SVR

28. You are transporting a patient on IABP therapy when you notice the appearance of rust colored flakes in the shuttle tubing. What does this symbolize?

a. The balloon has ruptured
b. More helium is needed
c. The IABP console has lost power
d. The patient has internal bleeding

29. During transport of a patient on IABP therapy you believe that the IABP position has migrated. Which of the following would be an indicator of migration that would support your claim?

a. Increase in UOP
b. Decrease in UOP
c. Decreased pulse to the right hand
d. Strong pulse to the right hand

30. You have arrived to transport a male patient on IABP support. You note the patient's cardiac rhythm upon assessment to be A Fib with RVR. What should be selected as the trigger of choice for IABP timing in this scenario?

    a. ECG trigger
    b. Paced trigger
    c. Pressure trigger
    d. Fiberoptic trigger

31. Which of the following conditions listed are contraindications to IABP therapy? [Select all that apply]

    a. Severe PVD
    b. Aortic insufficiency
    c. Aortic regurgitation
    d. Tricuspid stenosis

32. You are transporting a patient on Impella support. You note the power setting on the Impella controller is P-7. During your assessment you note a suction alarm. Which of the following is the best way to manage this alarm?

    a. Administer volume
    b. Decrease P-Level
    c. Increase P-Level
    d. Administer Norepinephrine

33. Which of the following Impella catheters are designed for use to decrease afterload of the right ventricle?

    a. Impella LD
    b. Impella CP
    c. Impella 2.5
    d. Impella RP

34. During the assessment of a patient on Impella 2.5 support you note a flat Motor Current waveform. Which of the following do you suspect? [Select all that apply]

    a. The purge fluid is high
    b. The patient sustained cardiac arrest
    c. The catheter has migrated
    d. This is a normal finding

35. The u/ml concentration of Heparin that must be added to create purge fluid is:

    a. 20 units/ ml
    b. 10 units/ml
    c. 25 units/ml
    d. 50 units/ml

36. You are managing a patient in the cath lab that has just been placed on Impella support. The patient now has a flat placement and pulsatility waveform. You note the patient is now in VF arrest. What is the most appropriate intervention?

    a. Start CPR
    b. Increase the Power level to P-8
    c. Turn the Impella console off
    d. Turn down Power level to P-2

37. Which of the following are key components of the Impella device? [Select all that apply]

    a. Controller
    b. Driveline
    c. Purge fluid
    d. Catheter

38. Which of the following is a contraindication to Impella support? [Select all that apply]

    a. Active bleeding
    b. Aortic insufficiency
    c. Right ventricular failure
    d. Left ventricular thrombi

39. You are managing a patient in the ICU that is receiving Impella support with an Impella CP. Upon your assessment you note a BP reflected on the controller of 69/40. Which of the following is true in relation to the BP that is reflected on the screen of the Impella controller?

    a. The BP is an unreliable measurement
    b. Hemorrhage is suspected
    c. The Power setting needs to be decreased
    d. The Power setting needs to be increased

40. During your management of a patient who is receiving Impella support, you recall that a target CVP for this patient is:

    a. >8 mmHg
    b. <10 mmHg
    c. >10 mmHg
    d. 15 mmHg

41. Which of the following is a cause for an incorrect placement alarm on the Impella device? [Select all that apply]

    a. Purge pressure is too high
    b. Catheter too far in the aorta
    c. Catheter is against the ventricle
    d. Cardiac arrest

42. You are called to the IFT of a patient who is currently on Impella support with an Impella LD. You recall that the console's battery power lasts approximately how long?

    a. 60 minutes
    b. 90 minutes
    c. 30 minutes
    d. 120 minutes

43. Which of the following is NOT a reason for LVAD placement?

    a. Bridge to transplant
    b. Bridge to Decision
    c. Heart failure
    d. Cor Pulmonale

44. During your assessment of a patient with an LVAD Heartmate III. You note what appears to be a "knocking" sound during auscultation of heart tones. What does this indicate?

    a. The patient is hypervolemic
    b. This is a normal finding
    c. The patient needs volume replacement
    d. Cardiac Output is optimal

45. The best way to obtain hemodynamic status of a patient with a LVAD placed is:

    a. Automated NIBP
    b. Manual NIBP
    c. Manual BP cuff with doppler
    d. Evaluation of radial pulse

46. Which of the following is a possible complication of long term LVAD therapy? [Select all that apply]

    a. Infection
    b. Thrombosis
    c. RV dysfunction
    d. Bleeding

47. The driveline of an LVAD is responsible for what vital function?

    a. Alarms
    b. Sends signal from controller to the implanted pump
    c. Connects the controller to the battery supply
    d. Provides pacemaker functionality

48. The output performance of a continuous flow LVAD is dependent upon what factors? [Select all that apply]

    a. Preload
    b. Pulsatility
    c. Afterload
    d. Set RPM upon implant

49. During your assessment of a patient with an implantable LVAD you note a "humming" sound upon auscultation of the heart. What does this most likely indicate?

    a. Hypervolemia
    b. Hypertension
    c. Volume replacement
    d. Normal operation

50. What would a "red" alarm on an implantable LVAD most likely indicate?

    a. The pump has stopped
    b. Device malfunction
    c. Low battery power
    d. Cardiac output is too high

51. Which of the following is a contraindication to ECMO therapy?

    a. Refractory hypoxemia
    b. Cardiogenic shock
    c. Morbid obesity
    d. Drowning

52. Which of the following is a mode of ECMO in which only one vein and one artery is cannulated?

    a. Phased array
    b. VAV (Veno Arterial Venous)
    c. VV (Veno Venous)
    d. VA (Veno Arterial)

53. Which of the following is a mode of ECMO in which only two veins are cannulated?

    a. VA (Veno Arterial)
    b. VV (Veno Venous)
    c. VAV (Veno Arterial Venous)
    d. VVA (Veno Venous Arterial)

54. An Avalon Catheter is used in ECMO in what mode configuration?

    a. VA (Veno Arterial)
    b. VV (Veno Venous)
    c. VAV (Veno Arterial Venous)
    d. VDA (Veno Ductus Arterial)

55. Upon assessment of a patient on VA ECMO, you note signs and symptoms of Harlequin Syndrome. Given your knowledge about ECMO, Harlequin Syndrome presents with which of the following presentations?

    a. Oxygenation in the upper extremities is worse than the lower extremities with adequate flows and optimal ventilator settings
    b. Oxygenation in the lower extremities is worse than in the upper extremities with adequate flows and optimal ventilator settings
    c. Cyanosis to the lower extremities due to distal limb ischemia
    d. Acrocyanosis

56. Which of the following is the primary role of the oxygenator on the ECMO circuit? [Select all that apply]

    a. Provides sweep gas
    b. Facilitates removal of CO_2
    c. Causes uptake of oxygen
    d. Provides augmentation of cardiac output

57. During the transport of a patient on VA ECMO, you note that the venous pressure drop is 345 mmHg. You also notice that the suction line is beginning to vibrate. What is the best treatment based on the above information? [Select all that apply]

    a. Increase ECMO flow RPM
    b. Administer diuretics
    c. Administer volume
    d. Decrease ECMO Flow

58. The most important action that can be done first in the event a patient is incidentally decannulated from ECMO is:

    a. Apply a tourniquet
    b. Clamp and kink the distal tubing
    c. Attempt to re insert the ECMO cannula
    d. Hold direct pressure on the site of bleeding

59. All of the strategies are appropriate in improving oxygenation of a patient on ECMO therapy except:

    a. Increase RPM flows
    b. Ensure sedation is adequate
    c. Utilize safe ventilator strategies (PEEP)
    d. Turn off sweep gas

60. During management of a patient on ECMO RPM flows should be maintained to at least what LPM target to avoid potential for clots to develop?

    a. 5 LPM
    b. 1 LPM
    c. 4 LPM
    d. 2 LPM

61. You are transporting a patient on VA ECMO. During your assessment of the circuit you note what appears to be clots developing in the oxygenator. You also note the patient's SpO_2 has started to decrease. What is the most appropriate action given the information above?

    a. Administer Heparin
    b. Change out the oxygenator
    c. Flush clots with normal saline
    d. Increase sweep gas

62. You are transporting a patient on VA ECMO and note the following ABG during transport.

pH: 7.17   PaCo2: 58 mmHg   HCO3: 23   PaO2: 400 mmHg

Given the above ABG, what adjustment if any should be made to the ECMO device assuming both ventilator and flow settings are optimal?

    a. Increase sweep gas
    b. Decrease sweep gas
    c. Decrease RPM flows
    d. Administer blood products

63. You are transporting a female patient on VA ECMO and note the following ABG during transport.

pH: 7.37   PaCo2: 33 mmHg   HCO3: 20   PaO2: 150 mmHg

Given the above ABG, what adjustment if any should be made? [Select all that apply]

   a. Increase PEEP on ventilator
   b. Increase RPM flows
   c. Decrease the sweep gas
   d. Ensure proper sedation

64. What is the maximum temperature that should not be exceeded on the ECMO heat exchanger?

   a. 37 C
   b. 38 C
   c. 36 C
   d. 39 C

65. All of the following are potential complications of ECMO therapy except: [Select all that apply]

   a. Anemia
   b. Hemorrhage
   c. Death
   d. Infection

66. During cannulation of VA ECMO, a small catheter may be used that bifurcates from the inlet cannula (arterial) and is pointed toward the lower extremity in an attempt to prevent limb ischemia. What is the name of this catheter?

   a. Oxygenation cannula
   b. Secondary cannula
   c. CRRT cannula
   d. Distal perfusion cannula

ANSWER KEY

1. B	34. B, C
2. D	35. D
3. A	36. D
4. C	37. A, C, D
5. D	38. A, B, D
6. A, B, C	39. A
7. A	40. C
8. B	41. B, C, D
9. C	42. A
10. A	43. D
11. C	44. C
12. C	45. C
13. A	46. A, B, C, D
14. C	47. B
15. B	48. A, C, D
16. A	49. D
17. A, B, C	50. A
18. C	51. C
19. B	52. D
20. D	53. B
21. C	54. B
22. A	55. A
23. C	56. A, B, C
24. A	57. C, D
25. C	58. B
26. D	59. D
27. C	60. D
28. A	61. B
29. B	62. A
30. C	63. A, B, D
31. A, B, C	64. A
32. A	65. A, B,C, D
33. D	66. D

REFERENCES

Abiomed Resources. (2020). Retrieved September 10, 2020, from
https://www.abiomed.us/educationdeck/abiomed-academy/

CENTRAL VENOUS/MIXED VENOUS OXYGEN SATURATION. (n.d.). Retrieved October 09,
2020, from https://www.lhsc.on.ca/critical-care-trauma-centre/central-
venous/mixed-venous-oxygen-saturation

Extracorporeal Life Support Organization - ECMO and ECLS. (2017). ELSO Guidelines.
Retrieved September 10, 2020, from
https://www.elso.org/Resources/Guidelines.aspx

Khan, T. (2020, May 05). Intra-Aortic Balloon Pump (IABP). Retrieved September 10, 2020,
from https://www.ncbi.nlm.nih.gov/books/NBK542233/

Kumar, R. (2020, April 04). What Is VA-ECMO? Retrieved October 09, 2020, from
https://rk.md/2019/what-is-ecmo/

LVAD Pics: https://www.nejm.org/doi/full/10.1056/nejmoa0909938
"Advanced Heart Failure Treated with Continuous-Flow Left Ventricular Assist Device

Medicine, M. (2016, November). Heart Mate 3 Pocket Controller Guide. Retrieved
November 28, 2020,
from http://www.med.umich.edu/1libr/CVC/VAD/HM3PocketController.pdf

Newcombe, V. (2016, November 27). Cardiac arrest on VV-ECMO. Retrieved October 09,
2020, from https://intensiveblog.com/cardiac-arrest-vv-ecmo/

Nickson, C., Frei, D., 3, D., & Nickson, D. (2020, February 03). Intra-Aortic Balloon Pump
Overview • LITFL • CCC Equipment. Retrieved October 09, 2020, from
https://litfl.com/intra-aortic-balloon-pump-ccc/

Nickson, D. (2019, April 22). Arterial line and Pressure Transducer • LITFL • CCC Equipment.
Retrieved September 10, 2020, from https://litfl.com/arterial-line-and-pressure-
transducer/

Nickson, D. (2019, June 17). Extracorporeal Membrane Oxygenation • LITFL • CCC.
Retrieved September 10, 2020, from https://litfl.com/ecmo-extra-corporeal-
membrane-oxygenation

Salim Rezaie, "Left Ventricular Assist Device", REBEL EM blog, May 29, 2014. Available at:
   https://rebelem.com/left-ventricular-assist-device/.

Ziccardi, M. (2020, April 27). Pulmonary Artery Catheterization. Retrieved September 16,
   2020, from https://www.ncbi.nlm.nih.gov/books/NBK482170

Made in United States
Cleveland, OH
26 May 2025

17229172R00062